The Wake Up Call

Cynthia D Kline

Dedicated to the reader of this book, and to the memory of a loved one who ignited my powers to be prepared for this inevitable loss, and to embrace the moments that are now etched into my mind.

Acknowledgments

Cover Art Design
Fabrice Berger-Remond
contact@ bergerremond.com

Edit Suggestions
Helping me collect thoughts.
Aimee Corser
Aimeecorser@hotmail.com

Cross country FT talks to keep me moving
forward.
Leslie Karzen
leslie@karzencreative.com

Contents

The direction of this story is about YOU,
the reader, who is like me, the writer.

I thought this wouldn't touch me.

I noticed a lot, but no one would agree, no
one would listen, or they would listen, but
they wouldn't acknowledge.
No Doctors, no specialists.
It was what it was.
This old guy has Dementia.
Good Luck, good riddance.

But… what do I do?
No help

You are on your own.
Even in the USA, this dreaded disease is
often undiagnosed. No medications, few
definitive tests.

It stabbed me in the heart,
Left me confused.

Left me without a home.

15 years of bliss.

A mundane existence on some days, yet one filled with love and laughter, adventure, and life.

Making memories.

It all goes by in a moment.

Did I cherish it?

It is hard to think of the way life was; it's like a blur, but I knew that I was content.

Maybe it's the trauma that makes you forget a little while you exist in a nightmare, but I hold on to the memories; I cherish them because I am the only one who can.

Fifteen years of bliss, followed by the dreadful...

DEMENTIA

Bliss...

*What a funny word, something you know
that occurred only when the moment
passed, but that is what it was.*

Until it wasn't.

Chapter One:

<small>◇◇◆◆◆◆◆◆◆◆◆◆◆◇◇</small>

'Rapid Advanced Declining Dementia'

That is what it was.

They diagnosed it as such.

The description is so accurate. It happened fast, with no time to adjust and no time to process. Just deterioration, quickly. A man disappearing before my eyes. How can I stop this from happening? I can't.

What is this?

A degenerative condition that worsens, in his case, almost daily, and is irreversible. In many instances, including Joseph's, it is a sudden cognitive decline. It had been approaching and masking as a bacterial INFECTION for two years before getting him admitted to the hospital and then released-antibiotics intravenously cured the culprit. Or did it?

The more it masked, the less time we had to act. We did not know. How could we?

Joseph, the most brilliant man I ever knew, with the most extensive vocabulary, now couldn't form a compound sentence. In fact, he couldn't form a fragment either.

He was a computer genius in his teens, building computers in the late 50s before anyone even had them. He built the first electric pinball for home use and coded before we knew what coding was. He was a child prodigy in electronics, then IT, and always in finance. He played poker for money at age fourteen, then he realized he could build a system of numbers to help with the tax system and became a CPA.

After entering Wharton College in Pennsylvania in the early sixties he stumbled upon his true heart's desire. He would be an entrepreneur, with no labels, no lane. He could be free.

In his youth, he attended a prestigious school in New York, Bronx Science, and his teen years were spent learning how to navigate the Science Research world and high-stakes mathematics. For an Aspergers-diagnosed person, this was a pleasure. School, his entire life.

He was in heaven. No need for sports- he wasn't coordinated enough for that, but give him numbers, give him science, and his mind exploded with utter genius.

Chapter Two:

❖❖❖❖❖❖❖❖❖❖❖❖❖

My Personal Einstein

He'd graduated from Wharton Business School and enjoyed being an entrepreneur for fifty-plus years in NYC, which he always referred to as the

"World's Capital City."

He had companies in natural resources, such as oil and coal; he bought and lost a gold mine in Colorado; he had shopping centers and large apartment complexes throughout the country. He built a gas line in Tunisia, and for fun, went on safari.

He did it all and in his own way.

This brilliant man.

This was a man who reveled in his ever-extensive vocabulary. He was a genius of words and phrases. He always used to say to me,

"The Road to Hell is paved with good intentions," and yes, he was often a bit crazy. He resembled a look like that of Einstein.

A character.

A memorable man who always got the best tables at the best restaurants. He ate at Gino's in New York daily until it closed and often popped over to the Four Seasons to close a business deal.

He was the quintessential 1980s success story in New York: a Park Avenue apartment, a driver, an office on Fifth Avenue, the 'de reiguer," no markings of the office, and the wife who was not exactly a trophy but thought she was and spent his money like a philanthropist without borders. She went to Africa to count the endangered species and to China to help with education. All the trappings of the world of the New York eighties.

That was all great until a major health scare- a bypass needed, and an irretrievable breakdown of a marriage. Too inconvenient for wifey to care for him, or visit. That was when Joseph decided enough money was truly more than enough and he relocated mainly to Fisher Island, Florida. At that time, the richest zip code area in the entire USA. And he, in his glory, was known to be one of the wealthiest business tycoons laying on his own private beach in a large beachside condo he had decided to ride out his bypass recuperation.

Fast Forward two decades later to me, the ever-present companion girlfriend, and a recent divorcee. I was not in the mood to ever meet any man again. I had been exiled to Miami Beach to ride out my years in comfort, graciously paid for my ex-husband who found his true love in a very young girl, younger than his own daughter. He was in heaven and wanted to do anything to rid himself of me for his new lavish life with his Babe from Eastern Europe.

So, my loving husband, now former husband, exiled me to Miami Florida, under the guise I knew people there.

I'd find a new life without him.

The introductions began. This was never my plan, but it seemed as if "it was raining men," and I found it kind of interesting, considering just how much I did not want a man; they arrived through introductions, on the street, at Gallery openings, cocktail parties.

That is when destiny stepped in and Joesph was introduced to me, by two separate introductions, both not knowing each other, but feeling two people like Joseph and me were put on earth to meet.

My final curtain was Joseph.

A gorgeous silky full head of wild white hair, a mustache neatly trimmed, and then as the years passed, he grew older but still quite the hipster, he adapted the track pants and polo shirt look with a track jacket replacing a blazer. In his later years, he became very 'Silicon Valley' look.

He was an overweight, brilliant, kind, respectful man who said he didn't want a girlfriend till he met me. We both didn't want each other, which magnetized the entire meeting and caused an explosion of interest. We had so much in common and spent every weekend together, talking, swimming in his pool, dining, and relating to a global lifestyle both of us had lived. It was thrilling on many levels.

As the years passed by quickly, we never intended to be together forever, we grew older, and we grew closer until I decided Miami life was too much CRAZY for me, and I moved on to a small coastal Village in California to live out the rest of my life in calm, quiet, and utter oblivion. It was a kind of Hollywood-style "closing the door". I couldn't have been happier. Until Joseph threatened me by telephone, he couldn't be without me and was leaving Florida to move to be with me. I didn't believe him until he showed up at my Montecito house with his little dog Harvey in tow. I mean, I call it a threat, but let's face it, that was one of the most romantic things that has ever happened to me; I felt like I was taking part in my own romantic comedy. The star of the show. He made me feel like that. His star.

Chapter Three:

Final 911 Call

Joseph was acting crazy, not making sense verbally, and very dizzy. I noticed him holding onto the wall with his hands, and not understanding where he was or where he wanted to be.

Feeling distressed, I walked over to him and put my hand on his lower back to guide him to the sofa.

"Sweety, let me help you…" I quietly said, acting in a calm but focused manner. I had a sickening feeling.

Joseph wasn't responding in any way.

He said nothing.

Sitting down, he stared at the wall, and I nervously stepped outside the apartment to call his Internist at UCLA Medical Center. I was worried and anxious; I knew Joseph wasn't right.

After leaving the obligatory message with the receptionist, his Dr called me back immediately.

She thought he sounded in distress; maybe he was having a stroke, or could it be another Bacterial infection? She instructed me to immediately call 911. He needed emergency intervention.

This was the beginning of his end.

And somewhere in all my Google research on his various conditions, I had a 'feeling.'

I knew my Boyfriend was disappearing before my eyes.

Chapter Four:

◇◦◇◈◈◈◈◈◈◈◈◈◈◈◈◈◈◦◇

Just an Infection

We both got older, yet felt young in mind and body, until the day I noticed his major IT skills, carrying two phones, always on two computers, dwindle to one. His Anger stemmed from the fact he knew; he knew but now could not remember. He struggled with not remembering and became angry, argumentative, and irritable. This had never been him before. He was generally sweet to me, easy to get along with, and happy to help in any way.

> *"Some people assume that aggressive behaviour is a symptom of dementia itself. It's important to see beyond the behaviour and think about what may be causing it. Aggression may be linked to the person's personality and behaviour before they developed dementia."*
> **(Alzheimers.org.uk)**

I believe, looking back, he knew something was wrong. He couldn't seem to navigate his favorite world of IT, and he became exasperated, annoyed, furious, and incensed at the smallest thing. He couldn't find his charger; he'd order three more – two for backups. He'd become irritated if the shower water wouldn't get hot fast enough, the upstairs apartment made too much noise, the avocadoes wouldn't ripen fast enough, the honey he liked in almost everything was too thick. He was exasperated and then irked nothing was working.

It was,

"The computer is screwed up! It's not working."

So, he would buy a new one, but then that wouldn't work.

"The operating system was off,"

"It's the password."

"The computers are all Chinese traps,"

The list goes on and on. There was always an excuse, a reason, it was always someone's fault, the anger and confusion not registering in his clever mind, he must find a reason.

"The keys got stuck."

"It erased documents."

On and on.

Excuses, excuses, and more excuses.

He even for a while stopped eating Chinese Food, he wasn't feeding into the culprits, not him.

He was suspect of Covid-19 origins.

"Maybe, my love, maybe…"

An iPhone, a Samsung, an LG. Tried them all, as he could buy whatever he wanted. I just watched in disbelief, but always felt that he knew best, he loved anything electronic, anything IT, anything complicated.

"NO!"

They didn't work either.

Wouldn't keep this contact list.

He said the phones erased his passwords.

Always a man with extensive and complicated mathematical complex passwords, remembered in a second, all gone from his brain, so he settled for only one.

I noticed this.

Looking back, I saw this change and thought it odd, but since I had no mathematical strengths, it seemed logical to me. How naïve, I should have known it to not be right, but hindsight is a funny thing, I guess.

He wanted to utilize anything new and innovative- a mobile secretary like Siri was new and exciting and he was going to use it to his advantage, but even that became difficult and mostly impossible for him.

"This Stupid Siri!". He would scream as he threw his phone down in frustration. It wouldn't text his verbal input, yet he never even spoke to Siri.

What the hell was happening?

He started struggling, slowly, slowly, for a couple of years, and then this….

Infections… or?

911 to Columbia Presbyterian in NYC, a hospital known for extensive research and the best Doctors.

This was, looking back at it, the beginning.

"Atrial Fib with a dash of forgetfulness," they said.

Really?

Forgetting?

From a man who never forgot anything?

It was during COVID-19, and the orders in the hospital were to treat asap, diagnose, and push the patient out as fast as possible.

Covid was worse than whatever he may have!

Looking back at the rapid diagnosis, it was always 'Bacterial Internal Infections' in unallocated areas.

What?

This was what they said at UCLA Hospital in LA, and in NYC too. Cat Scans and MRIs could never pinpoint where exactly the infection was. There was nothing else they could do. What else was there to do? What else was there to say? The doctors know best after all. So, it was back to 67th and Lex to the Upper East Side, New York City life in an apt where the new order of living was staying in. Sleeping in wasn't all that rare post-75 years old and Covid encouraged this reclusive lifestyle. A NYC kind of life. A remote life and a home office had just caught on in the USA and he was loving it. He didn't have to go out, ever. He loved NYC- you can get anything delivered, whenever you want. He was in his element.

I don't think anyone ever, at the time, thought of the dreaded word, DEMENTIA and no one even mentioned it. Whatever he said, everyone laughed and thought his eccentric style was charming. They said his extreme Asperger's was what made him who he was, eccentric, brilliant, and charismatic. These new behaviors were just part of who he was, they were of no concern.

And so, the story goes.

The NYC Atrial fib, which I told you about, the growing

"Dementia can affect a person's personality and habits."

older, slower, but still cognizant until that fatal day. To this day, people ask, did you notice anything in his speech, changed behaviors?

Yes, he did have a few changed behaviors that I recently recollected. He stopped talking as much, no diatribes, no rants, and often sentences just stopped, he'd comment,

"No Comment," or he'd kind of smile at me and say,

"Forget about this." Or

"It's not important". That was his go-to when he was obviously not remembering. He never said,

"I can't remember." Or

"It slipped my mind." Or

"What was I saying?"

Never.

I think this was because he almost always knew everything about everything, he lived a life of over eight decades with everyone commenting on his genius, his always top high scores on all his tests, which he never studied for. He had a photographic memory and was proud of that in that he rarely attended classes even in graduate school. He instead drove with a friend to Miami to lie on the beach. That was in the 1950s.

One time, I tested him on this theory of mine.
"What does a mascara cost in a typical drug store like CVS?" I thought he might not even know what Mascara is, but He quickly replied,

"About 10 dollars for the good ones." I smiled.

Correct.

He was almost always correct.

There really was no exact point of his no return. It was sudden, an extreme case of Rapid Declining Dementia.

Fast Forward to now, April 2023.

> "*Rapidly progressive dementias (RPDs) are dementias that progress quickly, typically over the course of weeks to months, but sometimes up to two to three years. RPDs are rare and often difficult to diagnose. Patients typically develop problems with their thinking, mood/personality/behaviour, ability to speak or understand, or ability to control their movements. Patients with non-curable forms of RPD may die within months or a few years from onset.*
>
> **(UCSF – Weill Institute for Neurosciences)**

He was rushed to Cedars Sinai Hospital in Los Angeles, and now, five months later, he's a vegetable of a man,

Not an ever-present Genius.

He remembers almost nothing, but he still remembers me.

He had landed forever in a Skilled Nursing Facility in Los Angeles, where he remains today, still somewhat confused as to where he is.

Some days he thinks it is a hotel room, a delusion I will not break as this thought is far better than his reality.

He recently told me via our Facetime calls,

"I am not fond of the room service here,"

I ask,

"What do you order?" Knowing this is all imaginary. He replies,

"Nothing much, a light lunch."

I smile knowing the days when we would go to Le Bilboquet in New York for their famous salads and a glass of sparkling water, or the years before when he lived on Fisher Island and we'd lunch at the Beach Club; he'd peruse the menu although he lunched out daily. He loved reading a good menu as much as a good novel. In later years, he'd google the restaurant to study its menu before he made a reservation. He was a New Yorker born of Parisian European parents and he knew good food, loved good food, and lived for the socialization of a meal with friends and family. A great pleasure he would be living and always stating this as such. He loved his life.

He loved the ease and flow of a life well situated with money.

In the last few months before his total mental collapse into dementia, he would be giving, it was his distinct pleasure. He was generous and happy in that state.

He loved to share what he had, always, until he had nothing.

Poverty and indigent living were something he could not at all relate to, and I feel this may have set his dementia into a spiral, knowing he was broke.

When the Dementia kicked in full tilt, the progression accelerating, no stopping it, everything appeared real, and I came to the sudden realization…

Picking up the shattered pieces is a delicate balance of lost love, and despicable detest.

How could the greatest guy do this to me?

Oh…Dementia…He's basically lost his mind.

Forget the Medical mumbo jumbo. He left himself broke, and me too.

No money for expensive lunches out, no money for rent.

He'd run his finances into the ground.

This guy left me alone, with no money. What an unfortunate set of circumstances.

Disarray- all his bills, past and present, no passwords, no records, no files.

Nothing!

Another sign?

Maybe this disorganization was him creeping into Dementia- a brain fog, a melting of his brilliant mind as we knew it.

Maybe this insidious disease was worming its way in for years. However, there never has been, up until now, any specific treatment to halt the disease.

No cure.

> *"If a person has sporadic CJD, their symptoms of dementia usually progress very quickly (within just a few weeks or months).*
>
> *There is currently no cure for CJD."*
>
> **(Alzheimer's Society)**

Only I ever suggested he had the dreaded Jakob-Creutzfeldt (CJD), and they still haven't. It's a human prion disorder- protein particles known as rapid progressive dementia.

Heaven help us.

Even his Neurologists at UCLA Medical Center never thought this was it.

Or never said so.

> *"Coffee drinking may be associated with a decreased risk of dementia/AD."*
>
> **(Marjo H Eskelinen, Miia Kivipelto)**

I can't help but laugh when I see research like this when you look for any means possible for a cure or something to slow down the rapid decrease of his mental state.

Joseph drank coffee every day of his life.

I guess this research didn't quite work for him.

He looked like an actor out of a Hollywood movie. An A-list celebrity. Everyone thought they either knew him or had seen him in a movie. and that was enough for people to remember him.

And that's how I'll choose to remember him, a beautiful mind.

Nothing more.

He was a walking kaleidoscope of thoughts.

I laughed at his endless approaches to a topic.

Never ever a dull moment.

Chapter Five:

<><><><><><><><><><><><><><><><>

Mathematical Genius

Financial Problems

I noticed this early on.

He was opposed to paying bills on time, in fact, he was opposed to paying any bills at all. He started saying,

"Oh, that doesn't need to be paid quite yet."

"That doesn't matter."

"They won't care."

"They don't know."

"I don't pay bills on the date they're asked for,"

Always another reason, another excuse. It was very disconcerting to watch someone who was always very, to the exact date, on time, and organized. He who had gotten, many years ago, a CPA along with an MBA, now does not care about paying bills, not care about paying anything. It was starting to frustrate me, but I was trying to keep him calm. This was all pre-hospitalization, Pre dementia diagnosis. Now looking back on this, I'm realizing, this financial breakdown was part of the breakdown in his mind. There was a point when he asked me if the calculator on my phone worked, I glanced up at him, thinking.

"What are you talking about? Why are you asking me for my phone?" I would think to myself,

"You always could do this in your mind," Yes, he was also a mathematical genius, part of the Asperger's syndrome, part of the autism spectrum that he lived on his whole 82 years meant that he was a mathematical genius who loved numbers, and now, he couldn't even use a calculator on his phone. He said it didn't work. He asked me to use my phone again and again and said my phone didn't work either. When I realized he didn't know what he was doing I would start to do it for him.

"No, you do it this way," I had an iPhone, and he always had an Android,

"Maybe that was the difference?" I thought. *"Maybe he really does know what he's doing, and I don't?"* I started to question myself because I was never a financial genius, I barely passed math and geometry when I was in the 10th grade. Although math was never the game, I always managed to surround myself with people who would help me in that area, and he was the one I turned to for 15 years of my life, now this.

He had absolutely no idea how to add, he had absolutely no idea how to use his calculator, and he had no idea how to use the phone. He couldn't even dial a phone number using numbers. It all became complete anomalies to him.

My heart stopped. My body froze.

"Something is seriously going wrong."

My beautiful genius of a boyfriend was losing all mental capacity. Right in front of my eyes. He had a brain that was disintegrating in front of me. There was a time when I realized that what was happening was definitely a mental issue, but I still could not believe it, I couldn't accept it. A genius of his caliber, my own personal Einstein, was beginning to sink lower and lower into the depths of not being able to express himself in the ways that he had before. Mathematical equations and mathematical business decisions were no longer anything he could do.

This is an absolute horror show.

A brain that was deteriorating in front of me. I don't even think he knew it at that time.

Fast forward to looking at him lying in the hospital bed. He had absolutely no idea, within a few days, why he was even in the hospital, he couldn't seem to wake up. The doctors took every test possible. What was happening? A brain scan? A brain bleed? Stroke? Cancer? Tumors?

Nothing.

Nothing showed up as positive.

My heart was sinking watching my beautiful, loving, brilliant boyfriend, lay like a dead person staring at the ceiling and reaching for my hand and saying nothing. This was hell, and I realized at that moment…

I had lost him.

The man I loved and admired for 15 years was now barely speaking. A grunt here. A yes there, mostly "no," his deep-set, beautiful blue eyes that were sinking deeper and deeper into his head, turning color to a deep dull blue instead of a blue that sparkled. He would hold onto my hand and say,

"Don't leave."

That's all he would say.

That's all he could say.

He ate nothing.

He said nothing.

He didn't move his body, just lay flat on his back, day after day, and his brain dissolved day after day.

I couldn't believe what was happening and I think now, I must have been in total shock.

Shock that anything could have happened so quickly. In a couple of days, he went from being one of the smartest humans I'd ever met to being childlike.

OK, so now what?

Chapter Six:

Legacy

I just cannot even fathom this man has left me with no money and a Trust account that was never funded. His credit cards that he always encouraged me to draw from weren't paid, overcharged, he has left me with nothing.

I'm in a position to file for Government Financial Help.

Oh, and guess what? I have been recently named in a business capacity to the Board of a Nasdaq Pharmaceutical Company. Yes, he co-founded a science-based research company that started years ago, and up until he had full-blown DEMENTIA, managed to get more money out of the company on loans than anyone else.

Yes, really.

A parting gift that means little.

Pays for nothing.

It's quite unusual for even Science Researchers to have this honor, but for a creative dreamer like me to be on the Litigation Committee of a Nasdaq Board is another twist in fate.

I can only smile at the absurdity of it all.

I promise to not forget your legacy, dear boyfriend, but puh-leeze…

He actually lost all his money long before anyone knew of his dementia. His life was a well-rehearsed script, which he performed daily. His phone calls and his Zoom calls were all business 24/7. But it was Monkey Business, and many people lost many dollars along his merry mental way. To this day, as he lies dying in end-stage Dementia in a care home for the destitute, he still believes he is rich. He lost everything and still has total faith that all is reversible with one business deal, although he will never again be in any business deal. He lost his ability to dial a cell phone, process a conversation, use a computer, and even recognize the people he had done business with for 40 years.

Finance was always his thing. He went to the University of Pennsylvania's Wharton School of Business and attended Bronx Science High School in New York as his High School and loved every minute of anything to do with numbers.

How could this end up being his downfall?

I was totally unprepared for any of this.

"ANY OF THIS!" I scream out loud. Only his little dog hears me. His little dog, which is now my little dog.

I've inherited his mess and a few of his pleasures.

How the Hell did this happen?

Had I really been living in LA LA Land?

YES, I had and was until the moment I came out of the stupor shock, realized the guy had left me homeless and penniless.

A Financial Idiot.

I have Financial Illiteracy Syndrome.

This is my **WAKE UP CALL.**

An Unprepared Patient who went into his state of Dementia, convincing many he was just 'slowing down a bit' at age eighty you would think this was the truth and that he deserved it and now we all recognize he was acting out a script for a life he once knew. Acting out through his dementia, covering his tracks as his mind deserted him. This is something I have come to find out is very common.

> *The older adult may believe that if they come up with excuses for their memory lapses, they might be able to convince others that all is well.*
>
> *Your loved one may start having what they call "senior moments" that increase in frequency and intensity.*

I feel he must have known it was coming on.

Or did he?

His doctors alluded to it, and he said,

"Absolutely not true."

Now, all the pieces of care for a dementia patient are left to the loved ones who counted on him, and all he professed, until he couldn't any longer.

I now MUST wake up and go forward with MY LIFE and without the Man and partner I spent 15 years within a dream state.

For the last few years, I have been Pre-Dementia Dreaming.

But no one knew it.

No one, not even me, ever wanted to think about it.

A time when all seemed possible, great, and alluringly happy for two older people who companioned gloriously.

BROKE!!

This man is now INDIGENT.

His Chase bank account has less than 100 Dollars.

What am I supposed to do with that!?

This was a man who at one time was a 'King' of New York- in the eighties when anything was possible with work and creativity. Yet another reason his dementia seemed so out of character, he was always a character and other top successful businessmen fell for his wit, his intelligence, mostly his known, big business deals. (Or were they really?) and his tendencies- smooth talking a la Bernie Madoff, we'll call him a mini Madoff for now.

He's now a dementia patient in a down-and-out skilled nursing facility in LA, and he still stands out. Even the various nurses find him funny, and handsome, and one even mentioned he was often charming between his bouts of anger. He's angry he cannot remember; of course he's angry! Wouldn't you be too? He must feel so confused all the time. He was so used to the finer things in life, and now look at him, he ran what was left of a business empire into the ground with this final stage of Rapid Decline Dementia. His last hurrah was with a tale of his Oil Producing Wells in TX as Collateral for several loans that were made by major Billionaires and long-time business acquaintances.

And now the tale digs deeper.

Rapid Decline Dementia, the end came crashing down.

Fast and furious.

Less than a few months crash, but then again this isn't totally unheard of.

All that 'seemed real' was, in fact, a delusion, but he could still hold that illusion up until a couple of months before he lost all contact with reality, he still could convince and charm, and he still could do a deal that would benefit him. Robbing others to entertain himself in a delusion. A delusion that no one knew of.

A personal loan from some of the wealthiest and most brilliant financiers. His reputation still preceded him…they required little in the way of collateral.

Now my back is against the wall.

My brain fog, going sober to the point I've little interest in anything except to save myself from destitution.

In Los Angeles alone there are over 75 thousand, and counting, homeless people, many of whom weren't homeless six months before. It's an epidemic created by a society that hasn't figured out what to do with high rentals, the cost of living soaring, people getting older, drug addicts with no extra cash, and being phased out of the working world.

It's a mess.

Chapter Seven:

∞◇◇◇◇◇◇◇◇◇◇◇◇◇◇◇◇◇◇◇∞

Dementia and Finances

Dementia can rear its head in finances, too. It will most probably break the bank, and dementia patients don't care. More than ever imagined, dementia patients, before diagnosis, start to do transactions, spending, buying, investing, etc. all in a secretive way- they are starting to lose the communication needed to actively participate in business, or even family finance and often present a paranoid, or argumentative manner to any questioning of their financial acuity. Remember, they are mostly angry; they have little memory left, and they know this on some level. They still want some sort of control.

This happened in my case.

The boyfriend spent all his money and fast- then he borrowed more- without me even knowing any of this. The Four years of this (Only figured this out recently and too late) constantly until he ended up where he is now.

Broke.

Totally indigent, and with Dementia- so actually he doesn't recognize this new state of financial loss. He actually states he is still rich, still respected, and can get 'money in' whenever he needs it. He is happy knowing this to be real. Of course, it isn't in any way slightly real, and showing him a bank statement means nothing. In the minds of dementia patients, they are what they were before Dementia wrecked any hope of reality.

Remember the 80s was his time of success. Anything one could imagine had a chance. This was a pre-cell phone era; this was charm and intelligence mixed with a bit of sociopathic brilliance.

Yup- you heard it here first.

Sociopath.

A Sociopathic Dementia Patient, and I believe this is a newly accepted form of dementia as we see it all around us. Politicians. Rulers. Big Business tycoons…Sociopathic tendencies. Charm the pants off anyone, and then a money grab you didn't see coming.

That would describe him.

And many others of his time.

Our former President of "Make America Great Again," Putin, Tycoons, other crazy World leaders of the day, all men, and often a woman or two thrown into this mix.

And the new world order as we know it gets juicier with fraud.

Sociopaths often rule groups of followers or admirers and the ones touched by dementia well....

Heaven help us all.

It is the...

WAKE UP CALL

Chapter Eight:

Wake Up Call

He actually forgot. He forgot!

Dementia takes no prisoners.

All is forgotten,

Or reimagined.

All.

He forgot how to walk, forgot how to navigate his body, and since he's lost most of his muscle strength, he is too weak to even try. So, the dementia patient sits on the floor, usually in their own urine as mostly they are all incontinent, or in a heap of weak body parts, and they wait until they are seen by an attendant or nurse to help them up. To pick them up from a total state of helplessness, never remembering how they ended up on the floor.

This is more than depressing if you are alone at home and have no help- which is what happened in my case.

He forgot how he landed on the floor and what he was even doing there. The calls made more often than not, the EMT workers who actually come in teams of 3 or more strong people to do the work you once tried to do on your own- which is physically impossible. I wish I had known this before I berated myself for trying and sometimes failing to help him. No wonder I'm not the person I was… my spirit has lost strength too- doing the impossible. Now the need for a Hospital, Skilled Nursing Facility, or Assisted skilled Living is a must!

And this is the dilemma.

I have no money - and past money can and probably will disqualify Joseph for Government or State help.

"WAKE UP CALL!"

No Money

Indigent

Loss of funds

Can this even be real?

Yes, it can, and it is.

Very Real, very sad, very tragic.

Being suddenly broke in America is a state I'd wish on no one. It's called Poor, or now financially deprived.

All your past glories are no more and basically count for nothing. In the case of Joseph and the skilled Nursing care, they act for little because of Medicare, and Medicaid. Medi-Cal etc. all look back at prospective patients' financial records to see what has passed in and out of their bank accounts, brokerage acts, etc. Nothing in your account ever guarantees every bit of Government and state help available. If one shows anything much in the way of all income, they are a target for the virtual denial process- info in, and immediately into the shredder. A death knoll for help.

On your own? If you are without, you're still on your own.

The Patient needing help is DENIED. Which is a word like a gut punch, a slit throat, a bullet in the head. It is as if the iron gates have fallen in front of me and padlocks have been put on.

"Access Denied"

"Sorry, we can't help you."

The shutters have been closed on my face.

It's Over, and Yes, you can APPEAL. (Another buzzword) but you'll need more money for an expert ELDER LAW ATTY to guide the application forward for your loved one in need. To do this on your own is quite difficult and in most cases impossible. Plus, it's more money out of your pocket.

Wake up as you'll need extra bucks in this form of medical help or intervention.

Personally, I've discussed this with various family members of loved ones who need financial help for their loved one, I've discussed this with many Attorneys and various Companies that actually specialize in this area of guiding the processing the general consensus is that there is help available but rarely for the educated, the rich, and the workers who paid high taxes years back, or the people like me. You really are on your own. You must find a secure source of help- and unfortunately, that doesn't exist.

"Wake Up Call!"

I'm unprepared, I do not have any personal extra money to help, and I do not know how to fill out the Government forms for filling; They fill me with dread and confusion, and I do not have the money to hire someone to do this. What a quagmire of confusion.

In Los Angeles, I found a few helpful companies- but be prepared as they are busy 24/7. In any case, you'll probably need help. And you will definitely need money- cash on hand to immediately pay upfront for services rendered.

It is just the way it is.

It is crazy because this is something that I never thought about and why would I when I had all the money I needed right at my fingertips, it is only now that I find myself in this state, broke and alone, that I realize how important it is to have money in this American society. You cannot do anything unless you have money, and now, I feel lost and overwhelmed, but I have no choice but to get this done, to fill in the paperwork, and to keep going.

Simply no choice.

Quitting is not an option.

I'm suggesting this because end-stage Dementia is very difficult to handle; no one knows the exact time frame of how long it'll last. Some say two years, and others say six months. It seems endless.

I could not personally help my loved one any longer- Physically, I'm not strong enough to pick up a man who has fallen on the floor and is dead weight, has no idea why he's even on the floor, and will not help you to get him off the floor. In a skilled nursing facility, they usually need 2-3 people of stature - nurses, aides, men who are aides, to do this same function, and it will happen in most cases- the falling- often as the patient has usually forgotten they cannot walk or stand, they don't even know they fell.

So, where do I stand?

I have no money.

I can't care for my boyfriend in our home any longer so I must find him a safe place to live, and for this I need money.

I have a boyfriend who needs me to fill out forms that I have no idea how to fill out so that he can be cared for.

I can get help to fill out these forms, but to get help, I need money.

I have no money.

Chapter Nine:

Am I In Hell?

Seeing him lying there in the hospital bed caused me to go into a state of shock; this was beyond anything I could have ever comprehended. He lay in his bed, not moving, barely breathing, not talking, just lying there like he had already given up. Eyes closed. It was a horrible sight to see, this once charismatic man just lying there, silenced. For the first few days, I would go diligently into his room, with strength, faith, and prayer, I would sit nervously by his side knowing, my love was about to die.

The interesting thing was that he really wasn't dying, he was in a deep coma-like sleep. He appeared dead. That's the state he would be in and out of for over a month. I would sit with him. Kiss his forehead. Hold his hand, even though he didn't hold mine. And wait, wait for any sign of the exuberant man that I used to know. Even a trickle of a smile, even a flicker of an eye.

Yet there was nothing.

I realized quickly that I had to take over everything now, he wasn't coming home, certainly not in the immediate near future. I understood that it was now my responsibility to pay our bills. Our landlord had been hounding us for rent as it was now overdue. I had been putting it off, hoping and praying for Joseph to wake and take back up his reins, but I had to accept that wasn't going to happen; I had to face reality. I would never have even thought of paying anything, other than my hairdresser. Joseph always paid all the bills.

Joseph paid for everything.

And I did everything for him.

With love.

With adoration.

As a partner in a great relationship does. Living together with this man who took care of everything was like a blessing.

It was fun.

Now, here I am standing over him in his hospital bed, realizing this wasn't going to end in a good way.

I don't know how I knew, but I observed him often, he didn't move, he didn't respond, and the nurses and doctors seemed not to care. I could feel my anger rising until I realized, they did care, there was just nothing they could do.

So, I begrudgingly, frightfully, accepted I was going to have to take over in most capacities. I am a very strong person but prefer to be pampered, and taken care of, it's always been my "natural state" that I'd lived in most of my adult life. I lived with elegance, ease, a lot of money, and a lot of access to every beauty treatment. Anything I wanted to buy, anywhere I wanted to go, the means were always handed over to me. It's not that I did anything for it really. Other than I never ask for anything.

It was a given.

Men would view me as very high maintenance and I never did anything to discourage this truth.

Yes, I am high maintenance, but I give what I get, I give the highest and I take the highest. Now I realize, my highest is fading into oblivion.

I called the bank number on the back of one of his credit cards that I used to pay for various things to see what the balance was in his account. The recorded announcement said.

"You are being connected to a bank representative."   Odd, I thought. When the bank representative got on the phone, she said,

"This account is overdrawn."

I sputtered. "What? That can't be."

I assumed that everything was there that was usually there. Plenty to pay for bills, plenty to pay for my hair, nails, and lunches out with my girlfriends in Sunset Plaza in West Hollywood. There was never a doubt of that, he would always say to me,

"Nothing to worry about, darling."

"I always take care of you because I love you. And you take care of me because you love me." We were happy. The representative got on the phone and said emphatically,

"This account is completely overdrawn. By several $1000." I went into an immediate shock. I kept saying that can't be. I know there was a deposit. I don't remember when, but I remember him telling me a couple of months ago. She said,

"Let me check. Yes, there was a deposit," she said, hesitating. "But that was quickly depleted," and she began to list the deductions one by one -all the checks that had been written, all the withdrawals that had been taken. There was nothing left. There was not enough left to pay the rent, the electricity, the water, the gas, the insurance, his health insurance, and mine. There was not enough to take our little Enzo dog to the vet for his shots, there was not enough to pay the maid or our handyman. There was not enough for Uber. There was not enough for food.

This man had left us completely and utterly broke.

This was, unfortunately, the fate that changed my life; this was my *Wake up Call.*

I was one of the women who enjoyed every day of my life with him, never questioning anything. I was living in a dream.

I was living with someone I adored, and I was living in my favorite world city, Los Angeles. Which is like a paradise for some people.

When you drink the water there, it's often said you fall under a spell. Not like a drug. It feels like you are on a different planet.

It's so beautiful.

It's so happy.

Every day there are blue skies and sunshine. People walk around in the most interesting forms of dress that they can possibly conjure in their minds, and it's accepted there. Every restaurant you go to for lunch is filled with beautiful people from all around the world and their beautiful dogs.

There is no age because everyone is in Peter Pan mode.

I felt like I was in heaven.

Now I realize I have just entered hell.

Being broke is Hades, a netherworld, an inferno of everything I detested.

Hell, what a perfect word.

You might wonder what hell looks like.

I know because I'm in it now. It's everything people have said it to be, and worse. All the people that you thought admired you, begin to avoid you. They're afraid you might ask them for money, therefore equating in their pea brain, you might want to borrow money, even family members react similarly.

You can't go out to lunch because you don't have a credit card. You can't pay your bills or rent because, first of all, it's illegal to bounce checks, and second, the credit card is so overdrawn it won't even take another charge. The cash machine knows all this and immediately blocks you, and cards are immediately denied. It's humiliating. You're bootlicking on your knees.

Once a queen.

Now a peasant.

Once the beauty, now a woman filled with disgrace. With An unflattering facial expression of utter and complete shock. It's a horrible state to be in. It brings you to your knees, you're now subservient, in a way, that's the direction only the mighty will fall.

Only the beautiful.

Your spirit begins to decay.

Do you want to know the most interesting part of realizing you're broke? Is that you must grab hold of whatever is left of your sanity, your creativity, your mental acuity, and go for it. It's a lot easier when you're younger, but when you're 70-plus years old, most doors are closed. Most people when you explain the truth will immediately back away. It's like they see you as a contagious, infectious, an easy to catch disease, and they want no part of you.

You have the plague- and that plague is called "broke."

They "lose" your number. It's humiliating. When not only you, but all the players in your life get a whiff of your broke status, they're in vanish mode.

They know when you say over and over again that you can't go on vacation with them, you're not going out to dinner, you don't enter Bergdorf's in NYC without a black Amex card.

Bye, Bye Darling - It's been good knowing you.

That's where I am now, except for the graciousness of my brother and his wife. I've retreated to their Cottage in the Woods to write this book, to regroup, and to renew my faith in myself. My other brother has been kind to me, too.

I will succeed.

I Can't go much lower; it's rock bottom here in hell, being broke.

The only way out is up.

Chapter Ten:

I Need a Job

I feel totally unprepared to enter the world again at this older age, it seems like a daunting task, and it's all because my Dementia Man lost it all; he lost his mind, and he lost his wealth. Yes, all his money. He screwed up every bill, every financial dealing, made enemies and all the while seduced me and the world into his charm of being. He was good at that, charming his way through life, he had that magical spell that enticed all around him, but it was all just smoke and mirrors. Dementia brought out his theatrical persona, I suppose. No one knew the confusion he was hiding because he hid it so well. That was until he collapsed and his whole world collapsed with him, as did mine. Unintentionally he left me to pick up the pieces of his life and try to rebuild mine. At an age where most people have either died or checked out of the working world. No less, not having worked a real job in over 25 years. My mind is in shock.

What can I say,

"I'm baaaaaaaack!" (With a throw-up of my hands into the air like I own the world)

I am up for the challenge, but a challenge it will be. With no new world skills, no new world ideas that play to an under-40 audience, and no new world appearance that entices anyone much now in this new world of half-naked reality. I have been catapulted into this world and I have no idea how to navigate it.

They actually say now,

"You're the shit."

I only recently realized that's a compliment.

I try to continue to go on, I have no other choice at the end of the day, with what little expertise I have, and write this book as an insider to a dirty secret world. The world of cognitive decline in a society that is also in decline. A society unprepared to help the needy.

BEWARE.

What you don't know might kill you, in this case, as when I realized the money that supported us was gone, as in totally gone, my shock and awe became apparent.

Or has it?

I'm unsure, it's hard to process.

My life has been turned on its head with no warning and I have no other choice but to take it on the chin and carry on. I need to find a way to not only support me and his little dog but to find a way to "be" an older single woman. What even is that?

Do you have a resume?

This is the question anyone will toss out before they ever want to meet you, Zoom with you, speak to you.

No, I don't.

And NO, I won't.

I was a Creative for over 30 years of my life, happily dabbling in all that dilettantes dabble in. Movie writing, projects like my

Cashmere T-shirt Idea- Propriety Privee, and movies that were bought as scripts and left to die on a shelf in a producer's morgue.

Hollyweeeeird games.

I'm too old for Hollywood now- ageism starts after one becomes 45- you're basically a dinosaur and that's the harsh reality of it. Put out to pasture.

Then, a rich man's wife a couple of times, and now finally a richer man's girlfriend, until the Dementia diagnosis. How can it go from extravagant meals in the poshest restaurants and sleeping in an apartment with silk sheets to heading directly into nursing care long term for poor people?

I understand many dementia patients lose their money, usually over a year or two with terrible business decisions, over-purchasing, blowing through the wad of cash they took out of the bank, and buying expensive items multiple times over, never to be used. I understand it is common.

I understand now.

Now it is too late.

Now it is done.

So yes, I need to get to work, and pronto!

As far as the employers see me now is that I am OLD, too old to be hired, too old to be of any real use to them, so what is really left for me?

Am I just a granny that's had too much filler? I still have a good face, not young, but acceptable, not totally ageless, but not as old as its chronological years own.

An attitude that can still rock a pair of jeans and look good, and an attitude that belies my broken interior.

Does my future look as bleak as it feels?

Or will this aging beauty be ruling the office of a creator's workspace?

Add it to the list of things to do.

Chapter Eleven:

Strength Training

He was so strong at one time. He had a great physique yet never went to the gym, "natural stone" he would say. His father died at 101 years old and could still run upstairs until the day he passed. His family always walked everywhere in NYC instead of taking a taxi. They would walk to dinner, walk to work daily; they would walk to their Synagogue every Shabbat week, and, when they went on vacations to Paris, they would stay at a hotel close to shops and restaurants so they could walk everywhere there too. It was a Family sport and an obsession with health.

He always seemed so viral and muscular. He liked to move boxes around the house, always noticing if I was watching him.

Guy Strength.

He had every tool to build things and fix things and was always offering others his skills. He once built a unit in the fifties to hold a TV, and that was when they weighed more than a small child. He built a wall in his bedroom to have an office space when he was just fourteen.

Illegal but ingenious.

Now? He is half the size he was - the shrinking man. He rarely moves in bed, where he resides most of the time, flat on his back or with his elbow behind his head, staring at the TV. He doesn't even use a remote now. He forgot how to use it several months back. I thought at first, he was joking around until I saw him staring at this black rectangle. It is the little things like that that hit me hard, you cannot fathom the thought of not being able to use a simple remote, but he couldn't. He almost forgot what the remote was for, not knowing where to push the 'on' button. I always stepped in, graceful but steady as I removed it from his shaking hand and put on the news for him, I never made it obvious what I was doing, it was just a silent observation that this was something I had to help him with now.

He loved world news and politics. He rarely watched anything but the News and Two and a Half Men with Charlie Sheen. That was it. He knew what he liked and was dedicated to those post-dinner times. 'His shows' as he referred to them. Daily, his shows became his only form of entertainment.

He would say he needed a little rest. That turned into all afternoon.

He would lament much, comment little, and then debate with me, the left vs. the right. He liked a moral stance, an objective yet fair politics in which the underdog got a chance and would argue their point. The needy lifted, and the conservatives stuck to the Constitution as written.

That was before the country took a tumble into socialists vs. racists, or so said the news. He was flummoxed at the sight and took to debate this seriously for as long as he could. Gradually, I noticed his interest was still on the News channels, but he couldn't seem to absorb what he was even watching and didn't really care.

He would then doze off.

Strength-wise, he was slumping into the sofa more by the day and couldn't seem to hold his body upright. Before, he had a very good, strong posture, and took it seriously. He didn't like slumping people, he told me once. He said they showed no confidence.

I would suggest we head to the bedroom and watch the rest of the news in bed, where he could get more comfortable. He always agreed, but he was getting too weak to even pick himself up off the sofa, and I wasn't strong enough to pull him up.

This was just the beginning of his waning strength.

He could barely walk but would refuse his cane and did not acknowledge he had a walker from last year's hospital stay.

"No, I am fine," he would say, "stop babying me." I couldn't stop, as I was afraid that he would fall.

I liked taking care of him.

I loved him.

Yes, I was seriously becoming afraid he'd fall, afraid he'd drop something and be upset with himself, afraid he would get lost in the apartment. I noticed he often looked lost. Confused. Like when I found him in the shower, just sitting on the shower bench staring. No water on, no clothes off. He said he had just showered. Which of course I knew was not the case. I tried to project calm, I couldn't show him that his actions were having such an effect on me, I couldn't show him I was worried, I tried to help him up, but he refused and said to hand him a towel as he needed to dry off.

He wasn't wet.

I found myself doing what he wanted, despite wanting to scream out, to cry out, but all I did was try to be calm in this ongoing insanity. This was before the diagnosis of dementia. Before we had a name for this craziness.

My tears fell quietly, I could never let him see.

My heart was breaking.

Chapter Twelve:

A Tough Decision

Why A Care Home?

Why Not His Home?

Friends keep asking me,

"Why did you leave him behind?"

"How could you leave him?"

"Why did you leave him?"

"What happened?" And each and every time it's like an arrow in my heart. Do they think that this is what I wanted to do? Do they think that I honestly had a choice? It's like my throat is being slit every time I hear their questions. It's the worst of the worst scenarios that I wouldn't wish on anyone.

I never ever would have left him alone. Never to this man.

Early in our relationship when we were both young and healthy, Joseph told me that when he was in his early 50s his then youngish mother, a Fashion Icon in NYC, a Beauty from Paris who reveled in the opulence of NYC Upper East Side living, made him and his father promise to her that she would never be taken to a nursing home, no matter what. She'd never be away from her beloved apartment in New York, which she'd decorated and curated to look like a Parisian palace in the sixteenth arrondissement where she grew up, and both Joseph and his father made that promise to her, with only the best heartfelt intentions to honor her wish. I, too felt Joseph and I had that same wish for each other. We would take care of each other in the very best way we could until 'Heavens Gates' opened.

Now, I live with this pain every day, knowing that I broke my promise to him, and all for the sake of money. I think of this daily, every hour, wishing things could have been different. I am always looking for a win, every lottery ticket I buy, every movie I write, praying for production, every prayer that I say daily, and I will never stop, so help me, Lord.

Never.

You could never know the pain and guilt that I feel every day unless you have lived through it.

If he hadn't have gone broke,

If he wasn't 82 and with Rapid Dementia,

If I had been an heiress or a trust fund baby,

If. If. If… and if I hadn't been completely at his financial whim, he would NOT be where he is living now.

If only.

But 'If only' is just a phrase, and if you live in these words your world will crumble around you, I must face the facts that my dreams and 'if only' fantasies are just that, fantasies, they are not my reality and I have to face up to that fact, regardless of how much it tears me apart.

I always say I loved being with him. I loved being his own personal courtesan, his muse. I was everything to him and he always wanted me with him. He didn't want me out of his sight. It wasn't an entrapment. It wasn't anything that was against my will. It was a delight. It was a joy. It was pure joy for me to spend 24/7 with a creative genius, someone who was international, someone who was handsome and doted on me and gave me everything I wanted, until the day he was broke, which is the day I realized, I had no proper home.

Without him, what did I have?

I was homeless. In America and all around the world, you know many people have no home, and have nowhere to go, just ordinary people who lived a type of life, and then that life vanished. It was erased because of one factor or another. So, this too is my factor. Call it fate.

When he was in the last days of his hospitalization at Cedars Sinai Medical Center in Los Angeles and I went to pay the rent for our apartment in West Hollywood, I discovered there was no money left. It was hard to believe at first. It was almost impossible to conceive, but it was real. Chase Bank had

$100 in his account. That's it. I was still in shock at his sudden rapid decline in dementia, which was breaking my heart, he could not speak, he could not move, he could not comprehend anything, and I was now facing the dilemma that there was also no money left to take care of him. There would be no apartment left in a few days when they evicted me, which they were already threatening to do since our rent was late and had already started the eviction process. I had to tell our maid, Emma, who took care of us, and someone I loved and adored, the truth. I don't want to lie so I must tell her that we are broke. I also had to tell our handyman, who came once a week not only to humor Joseph but to tinker around doing things that were probably not necessary but were enjoyable for Joseph at this stage of his life with no friends; He always said most of his friends were dead and his best friends were the handyman and me. I still remember the face, of Juan Carlos when I told him we couldn't afford him. He looked at me incredulously and asked,

"What do you mean?"

I didn't want to lie, so I told him the truth. Joseph had been living in a fantasyland and now was in the hospital with severe dementia. He had no idea what he had been doing for several months, none of us knew. Juan Carlos was in shock; I could see it written all over his face. He was not only the best handyman I had ever met, but one of the most soft-spoken, delightful Mexicans who I wished could be with us forever. Joseph always referred to Juan Carlos as his best friend and someone that he wished could move in with us when we bought our house and had a guest house on the property. He talked about this as though it was real to me, to Juan Carlos, and to anyone who would listen, and we did all listen because he had lived like this before in his past extravagant life. When he was a King of New York. Now, we had to let him go, and the guilt I felt for doing it ate me up inside.

Now, I'm realizing the misfortune that is real for Joseph and for me and Juan Carlos and for our maid, and for a lot of people who knew us, this misfortune was caused by a man who was a financial genius for many years of his life, had gone into total delusion. He probably had severe mental declines early before his hospitalization, but it had not been diagnosed. He had great doctors at UCLA Medical in Los Angeles, great Doctors at Columbia Cornell Medical in NYC, and also at Cedars Sinai in West Hollywood, CA, but not one diagnosed this. I feel that because of his eccentricities from his past, no one realized this horrible occurrence.

My friends told me to run.

Many said,

"You're not married to him. You don't owe him anything. Don't take on his debt. Don't take on anything. Get out of there now."

I couldn't do that. I loved this man for what he was and for how he had treated me for so many years of my life. The way he took care of me, always, helped me to realize the potential that I had, that many people had told me wasn't there. He let me believe things; yes, some may not have been true, and some were embellishments of his dementia, but even he didn't know that he was going into a sinkhole of mental cognitive decline and financial ruin.

As he lay in the hospital bed at Cedar Sinai Hospital, I knew that I physically could not take care of him. How could I? We were about to be homeless; I didn't have any help, I didn't have any strength left, and he was failing in every way possible; his body, his mind, everything.

I found him on the floor once. In the middle of the night. I tried to move him, but I couldn't shift his dead weight. It was from this point that I realized I couldn't do it on my own. I am 5' 7", 1/2, and 120 pounds, I'm not the biggest creature, I may look strong and yes, I look fit. Yes, I take care of myself, but, when I found him on the floor in the middle of the night, I knew that he needed more than I was capable of giving. Many physical impairments were starting that I could not help with, and I also realized I had no one to help me because I couldn't pay. In America, as we all know, everything is all about money.

Everything.

America is about the almighty dollar. Yes, Joseph had good insurance. Actually, very good insurance through the AARP and he had

Medicare and he had Social Security. But none of this was enough.

I had no money to pay for an apartment, utilities, nothing. I called every agency that I could have in Los Angeles from West Hollywood Family Services, Jewish Family Services, The US Government, Agency on Aging, Social Security, and Medicare for help. I called Various local non-profits, filled with the kindest social workers with nothing to offer but words of encouragement, all to no avail, there was no help available.

Nothing!

Because he got a Social Security check and had private extra health insurance, nothing more was available. Each and every day my heart sunk further knowing I didn't know what to do with this shell of a man. After Cedar Sinai Hospital pushed him out, which is what Medicare in the United States does after three to five days because they will pay no more and the hospitals are a money-making institution. He was med-i-vaned to California Rehab facility, on Century Park East in Los Angeles, which I felt at the time was a complete and utter joke. He had such high blood pressure it started to fail as they put him in bed at CA Rehab, and they immediately declared aloud,

"He needs to go back to Cedars Sinai Hospital immediately! We are NOT an Emergency Care Facility."

As I said, there was nothing to rehabilitate. They pounded his chest, called 911, and resuscitated him. Unbelievable! None of these Acute care centers or Rehab centers want a statistic in death. He has an advanced directive that states, 'Do Not Resuscitate', but they didn't bother to read it. They brought him back to this life.

As I walked around the halls of this new facility, I saw people on exercise bicycles, working with weights, and walking alongside a nurse aide. Up and down the halls, they walked. Joseph lay in his bed and stared out the window. The rooms were clean and modern, but they made it very clear he would be there only seven days and then Medicare would push him out.

"And what would happen next?" I asked in disbelief.

"That is up to you," they kept saying. The head of the business office there. Totally business-like.

"You can't just put a man out on the streets who can't walk, who can't talk, who can't fend for himself. This is unsafe." The woman looked at me and said,

"I'm sorry, Medicare will not pay, we need payment."

As I mentioned earlier, in this diatribe, we were broke. And so, all I could do was visualize my loving companion, Joseph, dropped off into the myriad of the thousands of people on the streets in Los Angeles. I envisioned him being pushed in a wheelchair to the curb and abandoned.

It was a hellish visualization.

It was like taking a hallucinogenic drug.

Nothing but an ongoing nightmare that I was living. This is the new America. Cities upon towns with the homeless, indigent, and ill, living on the streets, comparable to Bombay, like many other cities in the United States and around the world. If you have no money and you are a person of no means other than your Social Security, you're worth nothing. This was obscene. I could not physically take care of him. I explained this over and over to all the business heads of these institutions that were even attempting to take him in on his Medicare… we were homeless. We had lost our apartment because of his financial incapacity, and his cognitive decline. They would just say,

"I am so sorry, but this is our policy. We have no exceptions."

Then miraculously at the last second, I was told of an "available" bed for him at a place in Los Angeles called Kennedy Care Center. This is not a nursing home; this is a skilled nursing facility for post-hospitalization. An acute care facility is another name for this type of place. What I have learned about this type of facility is that it is a 'warehousing' for patients the hospitals can no longer help and won't. As most Americans use insurance or Medicare, which limits days paid for in the institution- and the patient of course rarely, if ever, has the thousands upon thousands of dollars in cash to self-pay. This is hard to fathom if you are NOT an American, or if you live in a country like the UK which has the NHS. If we need something, we need to be able to pay for it. There are no government-paid hospitalizations, doctors, or any help, even if you were a hard-working, tax-paying citizen for most of your life. Tough Luck. It does not exist.

There is something that is called "Long Term Health Care insurance" which many Americans apply for in their forties, while still working, paying monthly payment premiums so that when they are past 70 and usually retired, they will have paid into a company (all privately owned I might add) that will provide a bed, but this type of insurance is for high income earning people, and very few, if there is an underlying condition or problem, would ever qualify to get this type of insurance. Joseph did not buy this type of insurance. He truly believed he'd live till at least 100, like his mother did, as his dad did, and so did his grandparents.

The actual cost to self-pay for a Nursing home with any comfort, not to mention staff, would set you back around $12,000 and upwards, monthly. Yes–that's correct, over twelve grand per month. Hospital patients who are in an acute situation, meaning they cannot fend for themselves, they cannot care for themselves, are at the mercy of this. This was Joseph; not safe to be alone in this medical state of Dementia.

My heart is heavy as I write this, an injustice that I cannot solve alone. And my dear Joseph lies waiting in bed for his maker to call because I have no money to spring him free into what I know would be his happy place, being with me, and his little dog Enzo with a beautiful garden, and a helper for us.

Oh, and a glass of Lemonade iced tea.

That would be a pleasure for these, his final days. But because of money – only filthy lucre– we are not afforded that luxury.

I will forever feel a sense of helplessness and sadness because of this.

Many have said to me,

"You're doing the best you can for him."

Yes, that's true, but deep in my heart, I am devastated that this is all I can manage to do.

Whoever said anything about Life being fair? Not here in the USA these days.

"Equality and Fairness are essential".

Buddhism

Chapter Thirteen:

~~~◇◇◆◆◆◆◆◆◆◆◇◇~~~

Is This Home?

I went to visit HIM today in his indigent Lost Angeles Nursing Facility. This proud Man who grew up on the Upper East Side of New York, in a glorious apartment designed by his Parisian mother; with paintings, French furniture, Tromp L'oleil on the walls, and silk Persian carpets, now barely exists in a shared room with three dying men past 80, with nothing but a cot size bed and a memory that is failing him. One a homeless Russian, the other a big fat blimp of a naked guy with a continual blow torch style fan cooling his stomach. Long disgusting toenails poking out from the shrunken cheap bed sheets with no nurse to trim them. This is the Nursing home for the poor.

How the tables turn, how the mighty fall.

He smiles as I enter the room. He's so happy to see a familiar face,

"Hello, darling…"

With his once deep baritone voice, now barely a whisper, he reaches to hold my hand,

"You're so fine...You're the most beautiful thing I've ever seen."

My heart melts and just for a second it all seems real, like we have been transported back in time, like the man I fell in love with was finally back with me, but then it hits me, I am catapulted back to reality in a harsh rush as I remember he has no memory of me, of our life, of our love, he barely even knows my name.

"I'm surprised you're here." He asks me,

"Why?" I reply.

"I have a plane to catch to NYC, I have an appointment with my lawyers in 2 days about the divorce".

He says it with such conviction and a serious face, he believes it. That is his reality, he is living a delusion. I smile weakly down at him, while nodding my reply, I am getting used to his stories now, of the life he lives in his head, at first, they tore at my heart and made me angry but now, they are just a part of him.

I squeeze his hand and then my eyes dart down to his bed and to the paper bag that I brought him two weeks ago, just in case, filled with his track pants and polo shirts, never worn clothes that at this point would fall off his frail frame, it is now empty. Someone stole his last remaining wardrobe, from a Bottega Veneta bag I had used to place a change of clothes for him in. I guess even the Nursing home staff can recognize a BV bag.

He has nothing left.

Nothing.

From a man who bought whatever pleased him. He was addicted to shopping, a frequent buyer on Amazon Prime he couldn't even wait for the 2-day delivery he had to have it in one, like an addict, and is now left with nothing but the clothes on his back. He thinks the bag is his suitcase, his Tumi Luggage is no longer his priority. I notice he still has his watch on, although it hasn't been charged up in weeks. He loves that it takes his heart and blood pressure, he keeps tapping at it and informs me his blood pressure is perfect, he also says he no longer takes Blood Pressure meds, he's feeling fine. He's in great dementia spirit - nothing is real.

He's looking at my ass. His eyes are examining my body, I suppose some things never die. Guys got to be guys- thank the Lord. His sexuality is still evident- may be the last thing to go? His muscles are flabby and so, I assume, is his dick. Even on his seeming last days of cognizance, he's still all man. I laugh, it was one of the things I loved about him, about our relationship, the sexual chemistry was always on fire and so it seems, that part has yet to be forgotten.

"Still as great as ever," he comments, grinning that cheeky grin, his dark circled deep-set eyes, which used to be bright blue twinklers, now staring at my body. I know that he's not getting sexual, he's simply being the man he used to be, spinning the lines he always spun that would make me blush and laugh that bright happy laugh filled with promises. He's crazed now though, and I laugh with a heaviness.

He always charmed me both intellectually and physically, as a handsome, sexy, older man, my boyfriend. Yet now he is my patient who's beginning a decline into oblivion, sometimes referred to as early Hospice. My man is going down the rabbit hole too fast and I can't do anything to stop him. He looks at me, trying to say something, and then mutters,

"Never mind". He can remember less daily. He says, "Never mind" a lot now.

I tell him I'm leaving California, and he stares at me and says,

"Ok. Why?" with a look of confusion on his face. I tell him we cannot afford this place, I cannot find a job and need to go, but I'll FaceTime him, he says,

"Yes, do."

I say while holding his paper-thin hand,

"We had a great run,"

"It was better than great. It was perfect." He replies.

An arrow to my heart.

My tears flow, and I turn away.

Chapter Fourteen:

The NO Word.

"No, I won't get out of bed." He shouts at a young nurse's aide at his care facility. She looks bewildered and has no idea what to do. In many states, most of them in fact, have a three-time limit of asking the patient to do something, and then they stop. No Patient in California for example, can be forced to do anything. This is a skilled Nursing long-term care Facility, not a prison, and most certainly not a Lock Down Mental Facility. So, if a customer says "NO" they cannot, will not, and do not force them.

"NO!"

He doesn't want to eat, but he wants to place his food, (yes, it's HIS) nearby, within eyesight, with no plans to eat it, but only in the knowledge he owns it. It's a form of control as he has very little else in his possession.

This man had a permanent Amex Black Card—no limits on his spending, always on hand. He spent and accumulated doubles and backups of everything. Computers? He had five laptops. Printers, he had six, cell phones, he had all current new models, always about four, and backups that still would work if the sim cards were switched, at least fifteen. He had monitors for Zoom meetings, newly purchased that were never installed or hooked up to any power. He had every kind of file folder made, and a file holder to carry these files, although, he never put together any files once his dementia had started. I, as the Girlfriend, suspected he was a tad mad, a bit crazy, and a shopaholic. The ease of shopping with instant pleasure, no waiting times. Once he had Amazon PRIME, and his Credit Card was on his profile, he shopped daily, and as the dementia progressed, but still not diagnosed, he bought more multiples of things he didn't need, would never use, and already had stored multiples of.

I never knew much of this as he was still functioning, albeit a bit slower, he was about 80 when I realized he was slowing, and the Advanced Declining Rapid Dementia had not set in. Why would I think anything else was going on? He was aging, this is normal as you get older, right? You begin to forget things, your brain slows down, this happens to everyone, doesn't it? Dementia was something I never thought about, I never questioned, although I could see my man changing before my eyes, I had no idea how much he was vanishing, he was a life on its last legs.

When I might suggest calmly,

"Why do you need another HP Printer?"

"Because I want one." He'd profess and wink as if this was almost a joke.

He said,

"No!" often in those early days before his dementia diagnosis and decline. I often referred to him as cantankerous, and to our Spanish-speaking maid Emma, "Cascarabia" .... which means very ornery. He always, for many months before his diagnosis, would say the word no. NO to start a sentence because he was a complete control freak about everything, he said,

"No, that's not right, no that won't work, no I don't think so, no I don't care, no they're wrong, no they don't know how to do it," and so on and so on. I was starting to wonder why he always said no.

He used to be sweet to me all the time, and nasty or aloof in business to men who irritated him. Now, he has taken on this past behavior to all who would even slightly push him into doing something he didn't want to do.

"NO!" he shouts at the nurse's aide who wants to help him take a sponge bath.

"NO! I won't move!" he yells at the orderly trying to change his dirty sheets. Remember, this man was someone who insisted his bed sheets be changed three times a week, and at all the hotels he frequented in the world, daily.

The level of no self-care has gone even to his beard. He will not allow anyone to shave him. He looks like a dirty mountain man, and he knows it. He says he will shave, or he's got an appointment for a barber to shave him. Fantasy at best. An excuse so no one will touch him.

"NO! Get that damn razor away," He yells and points his finger, shaking with a tremor at the nurse's aide.

"I'll do it myself, later."

There is never a later, as he knows nothing of time now. Nothing.

This man was the best timekeeper. I'd always see him checking his watch, checking his cell phone time to compare, and then watching on the bottom of the TV screen to see if the times were all in sync.

He has no use for time now and is running out his own clock, I believe. He refuses most everything now and is waiting for God to call him home.

I discussed this NO word complex issue with a close girlfriend in Italy, whose 86-year-old husband with Dementia has recently started to use it too. She told me her husband, Alberto, would not take a shower.

"You're so lucky," I say. "Joseph won't even consider getting a sponge bath now." Joseph had always been an exceptionally clean man, always fresh breath, always neatly trimmed mustache, always fresh clothes. Her Alberto was the same.

We were both proud to show them off.

But that was many years ago. That is only a fading memory as we face our new reality and our new men. Now, both men in their eighties, with dementia rapidly declining, have only the NO word left as their power and their control. Nothing else in their life is their choice. They have no control over anything, including the decline of their minds. Everything else is decided by someone else, and in fact, I believe, this is killing them slowly. They realize they can't do too much, can't formulate opinions, can't put together a thought or even a short sentence, and sadly, both have chosen the shortest of power words, 'NO' to employ as their final sword, their combat mechanism.

We're broken at watching this demise, and we simply find disgust at the filth that they have become.

"Dear Lord, please step in."

My Italian girlfriend expresses the same feelings. If we don't laugh together at the chaos our lives have become, then we cry together. She always cries first- she's Italian, and I, the stoic, who's been holding it in, let the cascade of tears flow down my face. It's all too much, and it feels as if it is dragging on, even though, in the grand scheme of things, not much time has passed.

We both have developed eye bags and sad eyes.

Pathetic really.

This is from two women who relished their days of beauty.

It's the beginning of the end, that chapter of coupledom, talking about the men in our lives, the fun trips we took together, the meals, the holidays... It is really over now. We both know it, as close girlfriends do.

We're in agreement.

But in reality, it's not over completely as this insidious disease ravages our loved ones even further. Doctors have no idea when the body will shut down completely. So, all we can really do is wait and see, always hoping it's soon, but not wanting to lose them completely.

This always leaves us in a state of guilt. There's no cure, no stoppage of the mental state, although several promising medications are in the Pharma research trials for these men, it'll be too late.

Her Alberto still insists on driving through the winding roads of Rome. He was a Formula 1 race car driver in his twenties, and now over 60 years later, his mind frequently goes back to that time.

"A person with dementia often has damage to their short-term memory. The person may feel like they are living in the past because they're using older memories to fill in the gaps to make sense of the

"He'll get us killed," She screams laughing hysterically into the phone, "Or someone else."

"Take his keys away," I suggest knowing that is probably not the answer.

"He always has another set," she says, "and he hides them." She is scared, for good reason. We both know the outcome of this looks ominous. Alberto is insistent he drives; he has no valid driver's license and he doesn't care. She found him down the road at a cafe only last week.

"It's like being with a baby," She laments. "I Have to keep my eyes on him all the time."

I remember this state of being, the difference for me is that Joseph is cared for in a Los Angeles Nursing Facility. He tried only once to escape. He convinced a new young aide to help him dress and push his wheelchair to the Facility's front locked door. He was immediately pushed back to his room when he was told his driver hadn't arrived. All a delusion. Vinny, his New York Driver in the eighties, has been dead for over ten years. He was angry at me for days after saying I blocked his departure to the airport. This was heart-wrenching for me. The young aid knew no better. She actually believed him.

I was worried he'd fall, get lost in the apartment, walk out the door, and not know exactly where he was. Alberto is better off at home with her because they've always had their home outside of Rome. He's familiar with everything. Any move of an older dementia person is a recipe for serious disaster. Moving homes, and moving apartments all create a confusion they simply cannot deal with. This is what happened to us.

A move from New York to LA created a conundrum of confusion, both in apartment configuration, elevator nervousness, and in the end, him not wanting to even leave the apartment.

In New York, the building had an Elevator operator. In LA, the elevator had floor buttons that needed a push or two. Joseph couldn't remember that at the end of his apartment living. I found him outside of the elevator staring at it, not knowing what to do, what button to push, up or down. At the time I thought, and I hoped it was a momentary 'spacing out,' Which I sometimes do. Now I realize he was declining and seriously confused about where he was and how to do whatever it was he needed to do.

> *"A person who is time-shifted may seem to be experiencing a different reality to you. Try to remember that what they perceive is as real to them as your reality is to you.*
>
> *The person may not understand what more recent technology is or does. They may not recognize friends and family as they look now, expecting them to be much younger. They may think that people who have died are still alive. They may also not recognize themselves in a mirror, as they are expecting to see a much younger version of themselves."*

I found him in front of the microwave not having the slightest idea of what number of minutes to push to reheat his coffee. He'd stand there and tell me the microwave wasn't working.

I found him standing in front of the bedroom closet staring at his clothes, saying they all needed to be washed, and that they were there for the maid. We didn't have a maid, and the clothes were clean. His mind was mixing up reality.

> Dementia can affect a person's ability to remember how to do tasks, as well as whether to do them. They may struggle to carry out a sequence of activities in the right order, such as the steps needed to take a shower. Memory loss can also affect a person's ability to remember how to do tasks[1].
>
> ### (Alzheimers.org)

I found him at the sink looking in the mirror, wondering where to put his toothpaste. He'd been holding his electric toothbrush, not remembering to put the toothpaste on, and not knowing how to push the on button.

I found him in the guest powder room, looking through the drawers under the sink for his shaver. He insisted that's where he kept it. He'd rarely even walked into this bathroom before as he said it was too small for a man.

He'd always start my questioning what he was doing, with the word

"No, I'm here because of…"

"No, I'm not looking for the on switch," he insisted.

"No, I'm not taking a bath." He would state. But he never took a bath as long as I knew him. He always took showers. This was simply another place I'd find him running water and then forgetting he started the water. Once the bathtub overflowed, he said he didn't do it, he stated,

"I never use the bathtub; I'm a shower man."

If he wanted to get clean, he would declare,

"I'm going to take a shower." Then he'd shake his head.

"No," he'd say, "I don't need a shower." He shook his head over and over in exasperation as if he were trying to shake up his brain and put it back into place,

"I just took a shower," he'd state, as he sat on the shower bench fully clothed, watching the shower head drip.

He rarely wanted to even think of water touching him.

And this is another chapter to be told.

I'll call it...

NO WATER.

Chapter Fifteen:

No Water

He wanted no water touching him.

Ever.

He said repeatedly,

"I hate water."

"Hate, what about the water?" I asked.

"It feels hard, it's dirty water."

"Dirty?" I ask, hardly following this stream of thought.

"No, I didn't say dirty, but it feels dirty. Look where it's coming from."

I'm at a total loss now. I have little idea where he is going with this.

"Do you want me to wash your back?" I ask knowing this could be another land mine explosion.

"No, I do not," he sarcastically states. "I'm capable of washing my own back."

"Your hair smells," I tell him, point blank.

"You need to wash your hair."

He stares at me with a disgusted look.

"And you need to go to the hairdresser," He shoots back, knowing my hair is always a major thing for me.

I have to laugh; arguing in any sense with someone in cognitive decline is pointless because he never agrees with anyone or anything now. What's the point? Often, he has no memory of what he is arguing about. His reasoning now is almost always unreasonable and unwise. He can't remember even why he is making a decision.

His Dementia has accelerated.

We settle on nothing.

Again.

No shower, no help washing him, no shampoo, no shave. He's smelly and dirty now, and this once-clean man looks like he's homeless, and he doesn't really care.

"I don't smell anything," he says, looking at me in a way that indicates distrust.

"You do have a smell," I say, as he knows I can always smell almost anything.

"Well, that's your problem," he states, "you THINK there is a smell."

He's working himself up.

Stopping short, I disengage with him as it's known stress only exasperates this condition.

I guess it's another NO WATER Day.

It's apparent to me now that my dementia patient has no idea that the word no is nothing more than a different word than yes. He actually has no idea what he is saying yes to or no to; he has no idea of any consequence in the grand scheme of things, and that is how the financial mess that I've now found myself in came to be.

Chapter Sixteen:

Conversations

We are talking about random mundane things now; our conversations are not what they used to be. He falls asleep in between his comments, wakes, stares off, and falls asleep again, kind of like after a long discussion after a few glasses of wine… but this has been only a few minutes, and of course, he doesn't drink. It hurts me deeply as I look at him. I very much know that I have just about lost my best friend of the past 15 years. He is alive; I am talking to him, but I miss him.

How do you go about getting your head around that?

How do you miss someone that is right in front of you?

Unless you have stood where I stand now, would you know how that felt?

He wakes up and says,

"I'm getting a "Bridge" of $175 thousand in a week or so to pay off bills."

He believes this, and I almost do too, dementia at its best. It's like a game of make-believe, yet this is his reality. These are facts in his mind, but fiction in our reality. He talks incessantly about how he is getting a divorce so that we can marry. Another dementia delusion.

He has always been convincing.

Convincing, quiet assurance that all is good, all is right- right in the palm of his hands. Although all I can think of is how if this WERE true, I'd be able to buy my Porche, but at this moment, all I take are Ubers.

He's broke.

He has run what was left of his business into the ground.

This is Dementia ... a constant stream of irrelevant rants of some things that matter, and other things that don't, with a dose of personal silliness mixed in for good measure. Yes, he's still fun, and as he wakes again, as the man in the next bed begins a disgusting phlegm-filled barrage of loud coughing, he rolls his eyes and makes a face indicating his misanthropic self kicking in. I laugh; I love to see the small doses of the man that I adored still creep out to remind me he still exists. Barely, but he is there. Flickers of that man come through from time to time, just some reminders of that guy that captivated me and others, the same expressions, the same humor, the same cheeky smirk… yet what I see the most is the fading of a brilliant mind, he is now a man I do not recognize.

I remember how we'd often laugh a lot at the expense of people next to us, at restaurants, on airlines… our own world of crazy. Just two older people, completely, and utterly in love, who lost some years in dreams of grandeur based on years of past success.

Oh, how the mighty fall, and often fall together.

Chapter Seventeen:

At Least he Doesn't Know

If I can say much on this insidious disease, I can say that a person like him, living in this delusion, in his own little universe, is the best of all possible worlds, as he still believes all is fine in the world.

He is demented out and no longer has any interest in politics, which had been his diet of TV for most of the years I knew him. TV and News, 24/7, a background noise he felt would enter his brain. He loved every journalist, like Rachel Madow, Anderson Cooper, and Wolf Blitzer and he had an opinion to boot.

Now nothing- he stares at the screen- not processing anything going on.

"It can only get better and always does," he says with conviction. With his eternal optimism, he truly believed the world could only get better. He's said this the entire time I've known him. I on the other hand feel like slitting my wrist, but instead, I pray. I pray all day, for help, for patience, for guidance, as I honestly have no idea what's next. The thing that I know for certain is that his last days are being filled with positivity, charm, and he even still has moments of 'Master of the Universe'- although his millions are gone, and he is destitute.

I can no longer say I have hope in his dreams, but I am grateful he's still content, he told me so, just today. He said he's content, he has no regrets and entered his brain through a back channel. No joke- he felt background noise was monumental to his brain powers. Just as his afternoon napping sessions which he referred to as 'going to the office', meaning he went to sleep for 2 hours to solve a problem which he would then wake and say frequently,

"I have the answer! Eureka"

What a nut, I'd think until whatever he was mentally sleeping on, working on, came to be.

He was a sorcerer.

He is now a dementia patient.

If you ever meet a brilliant dreamer, I'd suggest you RUN, unless you can handle what I'm going through now.

Seeing the death of a dreamer before his days on earth are actually over, cuts you to the core. It's a horrid moment in time. Each and every time I go to 'that place' my brilliant dreamer is now a shadow of the prodigy person with whom I share nothing.

Because his all now is, NOTHING.

Nothing real.

Chapter Eighteen:

~◇◇◇◇◇◇◇◇◇◇◇◇◇◇◇◇◇~

Thinking about the Future

I'm actually getting my long hair cut tomorrow. Yes, I'm one of the older women who still have long streaked hair- because my man wanted it. Turned him on he said. If I can ever really imagine following Peter Pan again to his grave, I will have offered up my early burnout. It is tiring being a 24/7 girlfriend at an older age, and even more tiring, shall I say exhausting, that even face fillers can't help once you're past 70.

A month ago, I still felt sexy and young-Ish. A young-ish 70-year-old. Now I feel like I'm a clone of Methuselah, tortured by the early mental death of my best friend. I look depleted, I feel depleted, and my crow's feet are now permanently etched. Even Botox doesn't work.

He always said I was a Babe... me? Maybe then, certainly not now. How I long for those early days of our relationship.

Hahaha, I look in the mirror and see lines. It's interesting how the loss of a living lover with Dementia has turned my world inside out. No more dinners together. No more long drawn-out conversations until we both fell asleep.

I will visit him later in the day, post-haircut.

He says he wants to get back to NYC. He has basically no realistic ideas, nothing even remote. He can't walk; he can't even sit up in bed. He looks at me and sheepishly asks,

"Will you go with me?" Like the boyfriend from 15 years ago- always on his toes to please me, not sure what my answer might be.

"Yes, of course," I answer, and he closes his eyes and falls back to sleep with a smile.

I'm not sure what I'll do when this all comes to an end. Maybe I'll die before him. That's always a possibility. My mind wanders into this path frequently now and I know it's because I'm mourning a loss that hasn't totally ended. Joseph is still alive; he can still speak- not with the proficiency of before, but still says a comment or two. I do realize he has lost most of his vocabulary, but I can still make him comfortable speaking with me, and I no longer insist he finish a thought or a sentence as I did before his hospitalization because now, I know he simply cannot. Our relationship exists through Facetime. Funnily enough, we've entered the age of social media.

My tears are drying up as I need the energy to try to progress the little conversation we still have. I miss him so much that my heart aches. Yet, I am happy he still knows me, still likes me, and hopefully, still will smile, which up until now he does most of the time. I'm all he has now, and it's my obligation and commitment to him to try to be there for him while he still can speak. Many DEMENTIA patients stop speaking entirely, and I can see this is coming in the near future. If and when this happens, I will live this nightmare out.

Often, I imagine what it will be like when he no longer recognizes me or wants to look at me on Facetime calls. This is almost too much to bear, but I do know this may be around the corner.

Chapter Nineteen:

The Sudden Leave from LA

I stand over the bathroom sink, gripping the marble countertop, feeling like I am going to die. I am nauseous, I am weak, And I am shaking. My whole body is shaking. I am vomiting in a way that I have never imagined my body could convulse. This feels like every cell in my body is leaving. Every vibration that I've ever felt, every energy that I have ever experienced is departing my body all at once. I'm a shell of a person now, just like Joseph is a shell of a man. I'm leaving my man behind because I no longer have the capacity, the financial acuity, or the strength to care for him.

This is something unimaginable to me.

Yet it is happening.

I'm about to do something I swore to myself I would never do: leave someone when they need me the most.

Nevertheless, I have no other option; this is exactly what I am about to do.

My plane from Los Angeles is departing in four hours, heading back to the East Coast. I'm going to Pennsylvania, where I grew up, and I will be staying in a cottage in the woods. I'll be living at my brother and his wife's small cottage guest house. Here, I will try to renew, reset, and begin a new life without my partner, Joseph.

This is slowly killing me.

I will try to renew my entire being. This renaissance of me must take place or I will cease to exist. Quite honestly, there is a chance I will die.

I know deep in my heart that I will die sooner rather than later, not from illness, but from a broken heart, from doing something that is against every cell in my body, leaving someone to die alone. This is inconceivable.

This necessary move from Los Angeles happened suddenly when I came to the honest realization that there was no way I could afford to stay in my favorite US city. The City of Angels, and of delusional devils, which is part

117

of its charm. A city of dreamers that captivated me years ago. No way I could afford to take care of Joseph in the way that he would need, for the immediate needs he has now, and for the rest of his life here on earth.

I physically do not have the strength.

I financially do not have the means.

This is the sad truth.

I had spent the last couple of weeks looking at apartments so I could be close to him, so I could go to the nursing home and hold his hand, speak to him softly as he faded in and out. I soon realized this was impossible. Not only did I have very little money left to even survive on, but I also had no real job, nor any residuals coming in. Because of the position, and the financial state that he left us in, I had no money to get an apartment, little money to take Ubers and really no way to survive here in the short term. I had run the numbers so many times, there was no feasible way to make it work. First month, last month security, all the utilities, transportation, food, taking care of my little pooch. This feels impossible to me, and the worst part is, my soul and my conscience cannot believe what I am about to do.

This had been the implausible, the worst action I could take, but the only action that was open to me. I received an eviction notice. Nothing more to say really in a city where rents are astronomical, and the cost of living is at an all-time high. I had to go.

A revered LA Bishop and Friend in the LDS Church told me I had to go to save myself. I was drowning in sorrow and the inability to help Joseph. A Rabbi I met once suggested I join a temple prayer group. My strength was gone, I hadn't slept much in three months since he was taken away by the Emergency Medical Team in LA, and I had lost so much weight, I couldn't wear my jeans…they fell off me.

I was leaving my loved one in a nursing home, to go and live in the woods in a cottage, to reset my life. It is hard for my brain to comprehend that this will be happening in just four hours from now. I will be on an American Airlines flight back east. You might ask how I managed to get my airline ticket. I used the mileage that I had accumulated when I had my beautiful former husband and traveled constantly in the top tier way, first class on flatbed seats around the world. I always was a girl scout type- prepared as I could be. Always enough mileage for a plane ticket except this time, all my preparations were null and void. So, I made sure this ticket was first class, because that's how I roll in life. This too, was how Joseph went. This was our pact together, to live the best possible way we could – always.

This is how I will continue.

I lived in the very best and the highest luxury state that I could afford in the moment. I live with grace, I live with dignity, and now, I will live with a broken heart, probably for the rest of my life, knowing I did something that I think is incomprehensible to my senses. Heart crushing. Leaving my loved one behind. Leaving the man who had given me 15 years of intellectual brilliance, happiness, companionship, and yes, love.

I vowed to myself to never leave him, and now I am doing just that.

Will he miss me? Will he even realize as his memory fades that I am no longer holding his hand through this, his last earthly chapter? Will I be able to live with myself when this is over, and he is in heaven?

I swore I would never leave him.

I hold him in my thoughts, in my heart, and in my soul.

I will make sure that he is safe, and cared for, albeit in a Skilled Nursing Home, until the day that I can spring him out.

And if that never happens,

I will see him again. - it's our destiny.

Chapter Twenty:

Facetime

I still cannot get my head around the fact that I have come to realize the brilliance of our love is no more. It is nothing but a script now.

"Hello, darling". Always his first greeting.

BIG smile- recognition.

"Hello". I smile at him.

"How are you today?" I ask, already knowing his answer.

"I'm great. I feel super."

"You look good, but your beard needs a shave."

They don't shave him here in the home. The nurses fear that he'll pull away and get nicked, bleed, bleed too much, not heal, blah, blah, blah. It isn't him, I don't like it, but what can I do? So, I carry on like it doesn't upset me, the main thing that matters is that he sees me, he knows who I am and the sight of me has brought him pure joy. It always did, but now it hits me harder because the days that he remembers are numbered, the clock is ticking, and I will take anything that I can get.

Generally, it works like this.

I call into reception,

Then to the Charge Nurse Station…

Then the kiss-ass groveling begins.

"Please, could you, would you make a FaceTime call to Mr. Joseph?"

I miss him and since he has no visitors, I want him to see me.

"Ah, we're so busy, sorry. Can you call back in two hours?"

I call back.

"It's me again. Can I please get a FaceTime with him?"

"Yes, ok, ok," the nurse stands up, and I hear her speaking to other nurses, aids, whoever she needs to speak to on the floor on the way to his room.

"No, he can't go outside." She is probably referring to a patient who escaped his room.

"No, stop him, he'll fall."

I can only imagine who or what she is talking about.

"Excuse me, I'm sorry, I'm almost at his room."

I can see on her FaceTime she's entered his room. His measly, overcrowded room, complete with three men half-dressed, totally drugged up on anti-anxiety meds.

"You have a call," she tells him. "Would you like to speak?"

He smiles that big, dashing smile of his as she holds up the phone for him to view the screen.

"It's Miss Cynthia," she says with a slight wink. She knows he'll perk up with a phone call. Most of the patients simply wait around, lying in bed staring at a TV, and waiting to die. Some do die from a broken spirit, I mean, you would, wouldn't you? What kind of an ending to your magical life would that be?

"Hello, Darling." I see his face register pleasure and familiarity. I can't imagine what he's even thinking. I have no idea if he even truly remembers me or if I'm a memory from another life. He looks comfortable, but again, he's a good actor. He would have made a great Litigator in courtroom proceedings. He once told me he took the BAR exam and did very well but had no desire to be in a room full of men arguing their point. He said it wasn't creative enough for him.

My eyes tear up.

I wipe away a solitary tear with my finger and hope he doesn't see. He's squinting to even see me on her cell phone. But the nurse is a pro at this and moves closer to him; he smiles.

"Hi, sweet," I manage to hide my teary eyes; he looks so unkempt. His beard is scruffy, and he has a deep purple bruise on his shoulder and another on his neck.

"What's the bruise?" I ask into the phone, knowing he probably has not even seen it; the nurse answers,

"Purpura- a breakdown of inner membranes in the elderly. Purple Bluish tones on the skin surface and atrophied skin the color of purple. Forms under the skin, because the patient has a lack of movement, which causes this bluish-purple mottling condition of broken-down tissues, and weak muscles collapsing."

"We don't know. He has several bruises on his thigh, too. Show her your thigh," she barks at him.

He looks puzzled; she would have the audacity to ask him to strip on camera. This man is 82 and not into stripping or showing skin to anyone; he never has been and even in this new state, his morals are still high,

"I don't think so," he's adamant, "No, I will not!"

It's not particularly ugly; it's not even alarming. It's more just the elderly decay process.

Nothing new to report.

Nothing really said.

The nurse must get back to work now.

Another FaceTime call done. I got to see his face, and he got to see mine.

He smiled.

He remembers me. He still knows my face.

Chapter Twenty-One:

Mans Best Friend

The day Harvey, his previous Maltese passed away, was the first day that I ever saw Joseph cry. This was a day that we hoped would never happen. He decided he immediately had to get another dog in his life, he always told me that his favorite people were his pets. He had many acquaintances in the world, and an extensive phone contact list, but nothing and no one touched him like his beloved dogs. As a child, he had a pet rabbit, a pet parakeet, a pet French standard, a poodle dog that he was convinced his mother had put down at the vets because she didn't want him walking around her Parisian-style apartment and a pet pony. He detested riding but loved his pony, which he walked around in the country during the summers. Although he was an indulged child on the Upper East Side of New York, he was humble and never entitled. He believed that everything had its place, and all his pets were his brothers and sisters. Now, years later, he was alone. We were living in

Montecito, California at the time, and with the death of his beloved Maltese, who died in the middle of the night, he also faced the heartbreak and loss of his sister who died two days after suffering a stroke in New York, this truly was all too much for Joseph and he began to rely on me 24/7 and wanted me by his side always. He wanted his life to be family, his family, always. I began a search on Google for breeders that kept home breeding to one litter a year and found one in Burbank, CA. As we lived close to Burbank in Montecito, California, we were able to move quickly. We drove for an hour and a half for him to go and see if there was another pet Maltese that he might like. The breeder, Chris, brought out her two little boy pups, six weeks old and looking like two fat marshmallows, she put one on his lap, and the other on our driver's lap, who immediately peed all over the driver. We spent about an hour talking to the breeder about the Maltese breed. We took home the little boy pup on Joseph's lap.

Joseph named him Enzo Einstein. Enzo Ferrari the car he never had, and Einstein for his doppelganger. E2 for short, it was coined by our dear friend Jeff.

Now, Joesph is once again alone, without his beloved best friend, yet he never asks about him, he never mentions him, it is like little Enzo has been erased from his mind completely, and standing at the foot of his hospital bed, I soon realized that his bruising was caused by falling out of the bed, he could not remember this either. What does he remember? It feels like everything is falling apart and if this is the case, then maybe I shouldn't bring the subject up. Maybe the best thing to do would be to not talk about Enzo, so I never did. Now, five months later, with Joseph in the nursing care facility, never to return to us as a "family unit" I find myself telling little Enzo that I will never leave him, that he will never be an orphan, and that I will take care of him the best I can possibly do. I find myself doing things that I think mothers who are homeless or in poverty do, buy food for their pet or child as opposed to themselves.

I've never been thinner.

I notice now, when I'm grocery shopping, I would rather buy his hamburger meat than my food. It's really quite interesting and I'm sensing a side of a maternal me that never really had the chance to come out. I'm in love with this little dog and I've never been sadder. I've never been more loving in my entire life. I bathe him, I clean him, I walk him, I kiss his cheek, telling him he will never be alone. This little dog, who is now four years old, looks at me as if he knows what I'm saying, I'm quite sure he does.

He's lost his father and he never wants to lose me, his mother, and he never will. I would rather take care of him than anyone else in this world again. I thank God every day and every night when I get in bed and put him next to me on the bed. This beautiful little white silk-haired dog loves me like no one has ever loved me in my life. Just telling this story brings tears to my eyes. I never knew or imagined a love like this, but I am so grateful that I got to experience it.

I am in love with this little boy.

I reflect on the day at the breeders when we were asked if we were able to take him home that day, Chris, the breeder asked,

"Are you sure? Do you really feel that he's your little boy?" Joseph's eyes, fixated on this little bundle of joy said,

"Yes!"

Pulling a fat wad of cash from his pocket, his face lit up with a smile and his eyes shone like blue stars. He was again in happiness heaven, and we were soon on our way back to Montecito, California, to begin a new life as pet parents. From that moment, I realized what a wonderful father he would have made, what a wonderful mother I would have made, and what a wonderful family we could have had. That may not have been our destiny, but we did create our own little family, just two older people and a beautiful little furry white fluff ball, just like a little piece of cotton.

We were so happy.

Now? Only four years later, he doesn't remember this little bundle of joy that he adored so much. He never asks about Enzo; it's as though there is no past with him in it, and in some respects, for a Dementia patient, there is no past. He never asks about his little Enzo. He never questions anymore,

"Is Enzo OK?"

"Is Enzo sleeping?"

"Is Enzo in the pee pad area?"

That was all I used to hear, over and over, all day, every day, and now, nothing.

What happened to 'Man's best friend'?

He doesn't speak a word about his little boy Enzo. It is heartbreaking. His pets were his deepest love and yet now it is like they never existed. I found this very strange in the beginning, very unnerving, but at the same time, I thought that maybe his heart was so broken being away from us, me, and our little pup, that his brain blocked it out completely.

Chapter Twenty-Two:

〜◇◇◇◇◇◇◇◇◇◇◇◇◇〜

Forgetting Friends

I suggested a FaceTime call with his lawyer of 40 years. He always referred to him as,

"My best and only real friend," and for the time we were together, always smiled when his name came up in a conversation until… Lunch 2023. The lawyer knew he was in serious decline and knew this may be the very last time they see one another even if just on a screen, Ironically, when they started their professional relationship, cell phones were not in use. So, I was invited to lunch at the lawyer's home in Pittsburgh, all very casual, and simple and to merely touch base in this sad and awful long goodbye.

I call the Nursing Home Facility and beg, yes, literally beg for a charge nurse to walk to his room with her phone for the last goodbye of his lawyer- fifty years after their first hello. As the Nursing Care Facility is in Los Angeles, and we happen to be in Pennsylvania, the time difference is strained. The Nursing Facility is, as most places are in 2023, short-staffed. Stressed workers with no extra minutes for patient care let alone patient extra care with Zoom or FaceTime calls, remember this is a facility for Medicare patients. No extra frills. The Patients do not have a phone in their room, most have no cell phone, and in this case, my case, HE can't even hold the phone because his hand shakes, and he has lost all knowing of what to do with the actual cell phone- FaceTime works wonders.

The Nurse holds it up and he looks at the screen. Within weeks he has lost the ability to look at the screen without being told to do so. The Mega Man who always had two cell phones in his dress white shirt pocket, and a spare on his desk just in case. This was the man who 50 years ago in New York, paid ATT to install a line from this New Jersey Country weekend home to his home in New York City. This is the same man who has the old cell block style, called in those days a 'brick' as it did in fact resample a brick, in his chauffeur-driven Lincoln Town car- but of course that was the 70's and anything that could be paid for was considered a possibility. This was the man who had every phone call recorded just in case. This is the man who now lays in a bed in Los Angeles, not knowing where he is, or why, waiting to get back to NYC to do business. This is the man who now can't pick up a phone without dropping it out of his shaking hand.

My heart is breaking.

What has happened to him?

The FaceTime is now in motion. The Nurse is in his room, room 24-C. Which is the third bed next to the window. Ironically, he feels he's in a private room after having been in the middle bed weeks earlier.

A window seat.

I smile and look directly at the screen.

"Hi, sweets," I say and wait as he stares at me and then smiles back.

"Hi, Sweetheart," he says, smiling. He remembered me and his favorite greeting to me, the one he had used for the past fifteen years.

"I have Gregg here, remember Gregg, your lawyer?"

I question him in full anticipation of a happy reunion, or a hoped-for happy reunion, not expecting the blank stare, the unknowing look, the confusion in the moment.

"No, I don't recall," he says looking totally confused.

Gregg looks dejected but knows the drill. His own sister died from this horrible mental disease, he stays upbeat and smiles into the screen. He tried again.

"Remember we worked together, side by side for 45 years?" He says hopefully.

Silence, as my Love, the patient, looks blank. He has zero recognition and can't even muster up the strength to contemplate who this person was, his best friend, and trusted advisor. Someone whom he spoke to or of continually in the fifteen years I was his girlfriend.

"Remember, Murray, Samira, and Alice in the office?" He says hoping to trigger a long-lost memory.

My patient stares, and simply says,

"No, I don't remember."

Gregg abruptly leaves the room, as this tragically unfolding reality is almost too much to bear.

Our King of NYC is slowly exiting this stage. The last act is approaching, I can feel this in my soul.

The 'office' has closed.

His Atty Gregg is nowhere to be seen. He has moved on.

Bravo to him.

It is hard to see him not recognizing a man who had such influence on his life for such a long time, but I still hold on to these last moments of recognition with my love, I still hold my breath on whether he will do the same to me, I still relish his every word. His brilliant vocabulary is now reduced to a sentence or two he remembers.

"Hello, Darling…"

"You're so beautiful, darling".

"I miss you more than you know darling."

And when the FaceTime call is over in 2-3 minutes, he smiles when I say,

"Speak soon?"

He says, "Yes".

He no longer holds on to me, holds onto the conversation, no longer says,

"Don't hang up so soon."

He has no idea of what soon even means.

He lets go with a smile on his face.

Heartbreaking for me each and every call.

Chapter Twenty-Three:

Loose Ends

Friends come and go, we all know that, but interestingly at this end stage of dementia, even long forgotten in the mind's recesses, the sound of a familiar voice can resurrect a patient's memory. Joseph loved all religions. He studied religion as his minor at the University of Pennsylvania. I enlisted a Rabbi from Beverly Hills, a member of Chabad from West Hollywood, a Buddhist from my yoga class, and, I have an LDS outreach ward member go to visit my patient at his nursing long-term care facility. I also set up Zoom calls with a couple of old willing friends who want to say their own goodbyes, but my patient isn't ready yet for that. In fact, he seems to rally. A big smile comes across his face each and every time. Maybe somewhere in this deep memory, he feels the voices, he can hear the kindness now from the days of cutthroat business in New York, to now a fond memory.

"Remember your Assistant Samira?" one says trying to trigger a memory. "Remember how she always protected you from people like me?" he was an older ogre who lent this patient money that now will never be repaid.

"Remember how we went to lunch at, jeez, I can't even remember that restaurant's name, near Bloomingdales on Lexington." He grunts at his own memory lapse, and shouts, "That old small Italian joint and your mother was having lunch there the same day? Remember?" He urges.

He shakes his head part in irritation, but mostly in sadness. It seems unbelievable this Titan of New York 80's business remembers almost nothing.

My patient looks blankly at the Zoom Screen.

"It's not uncommon in the middle and later stages of Alzheimer's disease for people to lose the ability to remember and recognize others. Sometimes, this loss is limited to the inability to recall the name of the person or the exact relationship. A wife might accidentally call her son by her husband's name, or think that a regular caregiver is her daughter. A father might point to the picture of his daughter with affection but not be able to tell you what her name is.[2]

Other times, these changes are accompanied with anxiety, agitation, paranoia, delusions, and combativeness.[3] Some people have experienced their loved one yelling at them (the "stranger") to leave their house, or screaming and hitting them when they've tried to give them a hug because they don't recognize them anymore."

(verywellhealth.com)

"No, I'm afraid I don't," he says, with absolutely no recollection of lunches that were a daily thing, with almost always a few of the same people joining in. All are lost now.

The world too has changed, and those business lunches have become a rarity, but for these people, the distant memory of it is all they are lucky enough to still have. They're the ones whose brains still function.

The man looks dejected,

"Ah well…, it was fun".

"Remember, you had that corner table, and your own phone line installed there" He chuckles at the thought pre cell phones.

Another blank stare.

Nothing.

Chapter Twenty-Four:

Friendships Come and Often Leave

Ghosting.

As of lately, Joseph's been ghosted. He doesn't know this because he lies in a bed, in a nursing center facility, oblivious to all his friends. He used to have all the business contacts around the world that would call him, e-mail him, and text him up until four months ago, before his diagnosis. Now, he lies with the limited vocabulary he has, limited brain capacity, and eyes staring off to nowhere. The last time I saw him, I walked slowly into his room, which feels almost scary every time, like the unknown. I have a mask on; I take it off.

"Hi, sweetie," I say, trying to get him to recognize who I am. A big smile, as always, comes over his face.

"Hi, darling." He answers. "Hi, darling." That's all he can remember.

"How was your sleep?" I asked him. Getting closer to him so he can touch me, but he never reaches out to touch me anymore. He's alone now in his thoughts.

"Hi darling," I say again. And he parrots this back.

"Hi, darling."

Our conversations are now limited to a few words, mostly staring at each other. I try to think of things to say to him.

"So," I say, "your attorney, Gregg called you, but you didn't answer it."

He says alertly.

"I don't have a phone."

"Oh yeah," I laugh. I know he doesn't have a phone; I'm just trying to get him to engage.

"Anyway, he left a text on my phone," I say to him, "Would you like to call him now?" He looks at me, his eyes narrow.

"No." He says definitely, "NO! I don't want to talk to anyone."

"OK, sweetie, you don't have to talk to anyone you don't want to talk to, OK sweetie? Whom do you want to talk to?" I ask. His eyes narrow and close. This is a sign that he's either tired or refusing to answer. Then he opens his eyes and looks directly into my eyes.

"I don't want to talk to anyone," he says. "I'm done."

It's as if he knows his brain has stopped, his frustration waning. He wants to go home, I know this. Home to God. Home to where his parents are, in heaven. Home to where he can just stop this rat race that he's been doing for 82 years. My heart is broken. I know his choice is his choice, but I miss him already. I miss him every single day. I say to him,

"Would you like to call any of your friends? How about calling Les?" Les can still engage him in business, science, and research, Joseph likes him a lot. They love to debate business and science. Les would be a good mental stimulant for Joseph.

"Or would you like to talk to Bob?" Joseph felt that Bob was the savviest financial individual he knew, he admired him and had great respect for Bob's world contributions.

His eyes narrow again.

He didn't want to speak to anyone because he was finding it difficult, he knew something was happening to him and it was making him overwhelmed.

"Maybe tomorrow," he says. His Maybe tomorrow means never. He closes his eyes again.

"OK, sweetie, I'm going to go. I'll come back later." I'm going to go get a coffee around the corner from this place. His eyes open.

"OK, go get a coffee," he parrots. He really has no idea what he's saying, but he wants to be amenable, and he wants to be happy while I'm there, I know it. But I don't think he's happy. I don't think he's even depressed. I think he's just simply, done. He always used to want to talk to his friends and his friends called him from all around the world, several times a week. Right before he was taken into the hospital, I noticed that on the phone with whomever, he would be slightly quiet, as if he couldn't remember what he was talking about. One even asked him if there was something wrong? he would always say,

"No, I'm just tired, I'm really tired." they would call me after asking,

"Is there something wrong with Joseph? He seems different." I would pause and think to myself.

I think something is wrong, but nobody has made a diagnosis. They keep saying it's an infection and a bacterial infection in his stomach, a UTI, all of which seem meaningless. These were the doctors at UCLA. These were the doctors at Cedars Sinai in Los Angeles. Nothing showed up on any tests. Absolutely nothing. Even his brain capacity, though he was verbally tested, was still OK. And then, little by little, I noticed his massive vocabulary was dwindling. Each day, the sentences seem smaller, they seem shorter, they seem more succinct and more irritated.

When the phone would ring, I would say,

"Oh, it's so and so." And he would shake his head. He couldn't even think of the word no, so those friends would stop calling. It was as if each day, anyone who might have called him would never call again.

My heart was breaking for him.

Now, months in the hospital and permanently disconcert in a nursing care facility, he has no phone. The two cell phones that were always in the top pocket of his white button-down collar shirt during the week and polo shirt on the weekend are no longer. I canceled his Verizon bill and got rid of the phones. I got rid of everything, knowing that he would never, ever return to the apartment, and neither would I. As I watched his face on FaceTime later and in the hospital earlier on, I noticed that he had less and less interest in talking to anyone but me. He wouldn't engage with the doctors, he wouldn't engage with the nurses, he wouldn't engage with anyone. This was the person who for 81 and a half years of his life, did not stop talking. People would have to push to get him off the phone when they had only called to say a friendly hello, he loved to talk about everything from the news to the flowers to his swimming pool to his car, to what he was building, to what he was thinking of doing to one of the many, many businesses that he had entered. Now, nothing. Their hearts were broken just talking to their old friend, so they never called again.

It's very interesting to watch someone being ghosted by everyone they knew from the past other than the last person they knew, which is me. Even the family members, the far-away cousins, the old business secretaries, the maids, the drivers, and even his estranged wife barely called him. They couldn't bear to hear nothingness on the phone. They couldn't bother to FaceTime to look into his eyes which were now vacant. He was being ghosted by the entire planet. The planet he loved and the life he loved was now gone.

Now, he lay like a solid, bony skeletal man. A shell of a person just waiting for God to call him home.

I was his caregiver. And now? I am just an old memory, his very best confidant. His longtime girlfriend, now his power of attorney, his connection to everything else in the world he still exists in. I am left watching the person that I adored for 15 years slip away.

Never to return.

I noticed that I, too am being ghosted now. Too many of my close friends are tired of seeing me cry on FaceTime. Tired of hearing about something that the whole planet dreads? Loss of brain function. We are all getting older, and everyone knows this possibility may exist in their family. It may have already existed with their own parents. We are now of the elder generation. This is happening to the people they know around them. At least every person I know has someone they know, or a third party they know, with a brain disease.

We're frightened.

We're scared.

And so, they ghost me.

It is easier for them to block me out than to face my reality. They would rather pretend we don't exist.

Now, when I need friends and family to surround me and be close to me, to hold my hand as I watch my favorite person sink away. They stop calling me. It's as if people are afraid that this is contagious, that they can catch it over the phone. It's as if people might hear something that they don't want to hear. They can't face the worst of the worst, a brain loss, a friend like me, a good friend like me, having to go through such a trauma alone. They all know I'm alone, but still, it's too much for them to bear. I do understand this as it's very, very traumatic. This is what PTSD is all about. When my phone rings and I pick it up and it is a friend, I'm more than happy, but I find myself sinking. It is almost like a kind of guilt comes over me if I want to talk about him. They always say,

"How is Joseph? Have you talked to him recently?" I always say the same thing.

"He is slipping away."

They sheepishly ask,

"Does he recognize you?"

"Yes, he does recognize me." What they don't know is when he looks into my eyes, and I look into his eyes, the deep, soulful connection that we all know about, that we read about, that we feel, and some of us are lucky enough to have felt, is all we have left.

Chapter Twenty-Five:

Looping and Guilt

Guilt is another form of fear. Fear that one has not performed enough, that they haven't met the criteria of a good Caregiver.

A loving partner is no longer loving.

Yes, these are the pathways the brain goes looping into... round and round and round again. Tormenting yourself.

Looping is a term that really expresses this feeling as a caregiver and for me, the way out of this debilitating mental state is, yes, exercise. Walking daily as a meditation, no phones, no music, no partner, just walking, inhaling, and observing God's nature. Trees, flowers, and people.

I let the buildings kind of fade into a blur and try to stay in the moment.

Not thinking about what I plan to do as a caregiver later in the day, or in the next hour, not who I will call, or text.

Nothing.

Nothing.

Nothing.

Nothing.

Kind of a Zen state of nothingness, being in the moment and that's all.

This is hard to do for a control freak like me, an OCD person who has already lined up the chores of the day, but, taking a walk and staying in gratitude that I'm able to take a walk in a world where many can't do this simple pleasure, helps me to be a better person and a better caregiver, it gives me that well-needed space to just be.

Just walk.

Look straight ahead.

I become a 'Walking Prayer', speaking only to the Lord, and asking for strength.

I ask for calm.

I ask for help.

Thank the Lord.

Terminal Lucidity

He is, can I even utter these words?

CHEERFUL

This is a man whom I would never have used the word "cheerful" to describe him. Positive, yes. Hopeful, always, and anticipatory, continually. But CHEERFULL? Never.

He's now a picture of happy cheerful possibilities. He always told me his own father, when he was a small child, was worried he was depressed, he never smiled much and rarely laughed. Now he smiles every phone call and is literally the least complaining patient in a sad situation and institution that you could ever meet.

"How was your lunch? " I ask him, picturing the magnificence of our life when we first met, at clubs and 5-star restaurants in NYC and Fisher Island off Miami where he lived for many years in expensive bliss.

"Wonderful!" He answers with a smile. He appreciates every fresh morsel of food. Except there is never anything on his plastic tray that is fresh.

Never.

It's Jello in a plastic cup, unrecognizable stew, no salt, which he loved, no sliced cucumbers and radishes which he requested, and no fresh avocados and tomatoes which were his daily snack. This is all basically a mush of unrecognizable, easy-to-eat and swallow food that if he were not in a cognitive state, he would never even give to the garbage without complaining.

Now he says,

"Very good food here."

I'm stunned, but say nothing, because these days, he rarely eats anything, so anything he does eat is good!

He's in a continual "NO" phase.

NO to any food or drink most of the time, although I did notice he ate the special July 4th holiday meal of an American cheeseburger, French fries, and a cookie. He remarked it was so delicious. This struck me as odd because in fifteen years I have never once seen him eat a hamburger, cheeseburger, or anything similar. His favorite 'cheat meal' as he called it was the Hebrew National Jumbo Hotdog. Only one, on a plate, no bun, with a touch of mustard.

Never a Hamburger.

He's lost a great deal of weight, and most of any muscle he had. He hasn't walked in months and hasn't gotten out of bed either.

Terminal Lucidity is often a wish gone viral.

What I mean by that is, when the patient seems like a comeback from the dead has occurred, the caregiver rushes to text, email, and declare,

"I can't believe I'm saying this…but"

The comeback is a momentary uplift at the beginning of the near end, the pre-death state where the patient seems to have a few last-minute regrets, needs closure and wants to say goodbyes.

It is momentary.

Chapter Twenty-Six:

You Don't Know

What You Don't Know

I guess my life has changed substantially in the last few months; I live my life day to day, not really thinking much about my next steps, just trying to survive and trying to get through each day. Someone asked me recently,

"So, what do you do with your days, now that Joseph is in a home?"

What do I do with my days?

Hmm.

It made me think,

I don't know,

What I now do daily is… Well…

You don't know what you don't know. That's what I've been finding out ever since Joseph entered a Los Angeles Critical Acute care facility. I had no idea of the complications of the legalities; I'm his Power of Attorney, the financial needs. What it will take to keep him inside and safe, secure, and cared for is my responsibility. I had always thought that as we grew older together, I would be the caretaker for him and his money would pay for all the help, the home, and the needs that we would have. It's not that we lived a simple life, but our needs and wants were rather simple in comparison to our neighbors in Los Angeles, the home of glitz and glam and Hollywood. A place that I loved for 40 years of my life that felt very comfortable and very secure in. It was safe and Beverly Hills, where I lived for most of this time, felt like a neighborhood of happy people. I was one of them. It mirrored even the simplicity of the life that I was living. Now it's often referred to as quiet luxury.

But now everything has changed.

Everything.

So, you might wonder, what is it that you do during the day now?

Post 70 years old.

My companion of 15 years whose brain has melted into total dementia is now living in a Nursing Care Facility and indigent. But I have already admitted to you this new state of being.

I wake up in the morning, and I immediately start to pray.

I pray, I meditate, and I plan.

Praying is something I've always done my entire life, but now I'm praying for my survival. I'm praying to be kept off the streets, praying I'm not thrown into the homeless society that has taken over cities across America with people like me, who have suddenly fallen on hard times in an ever-increasing costly life of inflation. The Government spending has only added to the rising costs of everything. The rent for a studio apartment in any major city now is over one thousand dollars.

I'm praying that the creativity that I know I have in every form, whether it be writing, painting, or thinking; the creativity that people have TOLD me my entire life is who I am, is within me ready to manifest. That it will help me in my time of need, I must survive, and my creativity will keep me off the streets, I know it will, I can feel it rooted in these worn bones of mine, my time is still coming. This is just the closing of a chapter and not of a book.

I grew up in a very gilded environment in the '50s. Everything I wanted I was given. Not spoiled, but I had a father who indulged me and a mother who adored me, and now I have no one. I have nothing. Joseph indulged me daily, he once told me,

"There is Nothing...", he said, and looked deep into my eyes in his doorway as I went to the spa on Fisher Island, "Nothing, I would deny you."

I have Joseph's little dog, Enzo, my constant companion, and inspiration for us to survive. When walking around the streets of Los Angeles down near the downtown museums, I saw two homeless encampments, people living in makeshift tents of cardboard, old construction plastic tarps, dilapidated tossed-out mover's boxes, and the like. Constructions created from materials everyone else would throw out, dotted on sidewalks, thousands upon thousands of people, some drug addicts, most others leveled to live a life of misfortune that I vowed to never succumb to.

So, you ask, what is it that I do? Now that Joseph and I no longer live together, and I'm on my own, what is my daily schedule?

Do I even have a routine?

Yes, I do.

I have always had a routine, and always will.

I drink my morning coffee, but no longer make his, although I sometimes find myself going to reach for two cups, forgetting I only need one. I still always make my bed; I no longer have a maid. After doing my yoga every morning and after taking my walk when the weather is pleasant wherever I am, I meditate, and I pray.

I pray that God gives me the grace to get through this unscathed.

Lately, the biggest challenge that I have is the challenge that I never wanted to face, and that is bureaucracy. Government bureaucracy.

State bureaucracy. In this case, medical insurance companies, Medi-Cal, Medicare, and the like.

Bureaucracy all day, every day.

Typical that someone like me, who has very limited knowledge of legal, accounting, mathematical, or even day-to-day realistic business experience, I basically am clueless, has got to face these hurdles. I lived a pampered life, I was mostly taken care of by my lovers, husbands, and now…I must step up to the plate, and care for this man who cared for me for 15 years. I have no other option, no other choice. He depends on me, and I depend on myself. It is the least I can do for a man who took care of me for such a long time. A man who not only indulged me but looked after my needs.

This is my goal daily.

This is my responsibility daily.

I am the only advocate he has.

Today, I will spend the day trying to figure out what Medi-Cal will offer up. This I learned, is the Medicare component of the state of California, hopefully, it will kick in and give financial help to offset Joseph's Social Security monthly payments. His monthly allotments from the government are not enough. Interestingly, he has a top-tier Social Security payment, which means a lot of $$$, but not enough for his care. The USA really has no care for people who have spent their lives working and paying taxes only to be left when the hard times come. When they have fallen.

Sad but true and it doesn't look like it is changing anytime soon.

Financially, to care for him in a Skilled Care Nursing Facility in Los Angeles, which is substandard, with three men in a room, no fresh food, very little health care, and little compassion, is expensive! This is basic care, no extra comforts, comforts that he has long become accustomed to, they aren't here. He is getting the care of an indigent; this is where he lives now, and even though he seems to not be fazed by his new living standards, I am! But I don't have any way to make it better for him, I can't pay for anything better for him. There is no help on the telephone from the facility, they do not offer any support. Maybe it is because I live thousands of miles away, but again, there is nothing I can do about that either. If I could have stayed close to Joseph, I would in a heartbeat, but instead, I'm here, thousands of miles away in a guest cottage that my dear brother and his wonderful wife have given me to live in while I figure out my life and the life that I will try to create for Joseph until God calls him home.

This is what I do daily.

I had never envisioned this kind of life. What I had envisioned for Joseph and me was a home in Beverly Hills, Gurlee, as my constant companion live-in maid, a pool, and a lounge chair where he could sit. We would live out our years in a beautiful garden. I knew that he would probably never go into his beloved swimming pool again, he couldn't walk, he can barely stand, but I could sit with him and hold his hand and let him live in a paradise of sunshine, warm weather, and quiet. In a visual paradise, a small garden is what I envisioned, with two lounge chairs a table, and two lemonades, nothing more.

I sometimes daydream about the life I envisioned for us, wishing things were the way I could see them in my head, but it doesn't do any good to dwell on the 'what-ifs' of life. We couldn't even have this now as this is the 'American dream' post-Joseph's financial fall into poverty.

This is America now.

A paradise reserved for the very rich. No longer reachable even for the masses that were once called the middle class.

Yes, Los Angeles to us is the most beautiful paradise left in the world.

Now, my new norm is scrapping to simply get by. Inflation has risen in the past few months and even though I am a frugal person, getting by with just the skin of my teeth is not an option, it's a reality. A reality I never once thought would be mine, but it is, unbelievably. As I peruse my clothes, shoes, and bags, all my past spoils of a life lived in luxury I can only imagine I must have been nuts to buy all this material accouterment, things that now no longer serve me. Even on a recent visit to a consignment shop, I was told,

"No one buys things this elegant now" the shopkeeper stated matter of fact.

"We sell athletic leisure things." She looks at me with disdain.

All around me, businesses are having trouble surviving post-pandemic, vacant office buildings, homes too expensive stay unsold, and ones too cheap are left to fall apart, including skilled nursing home facilities, and facilities like the one Joseph resides in now. It needs a new front door with a security system, among many other things, it looks tired and old mimicking the residents that reside there. Money has become a huge issue.

And so what? You might say. What do I do every day? I told you earlier in this book, that getting a job past the age of 70 in the United States is close to impossible, if not impossible. The care work that I was always doing as a companion for my boyfriend Joseph was my "job" and I loved it. I've always loved being needed in every marriage that I've ever had and every relationship that I've ever had. I find that I'm a person who enjoys caretaking. Joseph always referred to me as his Courtesan. I entertained him. I enjoy being the cook, I enjoy being the confidant, and I enjoy being the conversationalist. I enjoy planning the day for myself and my loved ones, and now this job has been taken from me.

And so, as I write this, you may ask, what is it that you *actually* do?

Besides the actual horror of trying to keep Joseph in a Facility to care for him, because of money, and filthy lucre, I meditate the day away.

One day, if only…
Oh, and ….

I have a tomato plant that has three tomatoes on it, they're cherry tomatoes. Someone gave it to me as a small plant and I put it out in the sun, and it's been growing daily, every day when I look at this plant I see an infinitesimal amount of growth, I see this as a metaphor for me, I'm actually living a life of growth at this stage, how many people my age or older have stopped? This is the time in your life when you should be slowing down and settling. Some have retired to hit golf balls, some play cards, some have made the TV news their all-consuming reality, some go on cruises, and then there's the rest of us, the creatives, the musicians, the writers, the dancers, the artists. We continue in an ageless format. We've forgotten that we are as old as we are and the only thing that hasn't been forgotten are the weekly forms that I have to fill out for Joseph. He's 82, he can no longer read, no longer write, no longer process much more than a few words, and can no longer sign his name. It is clear he is nearing his final days here on Earth. Kind of makes me laugh when I think about it. He had the worst handwriting, and his signature was always just a scribble, but it was his signature and I loved it. He said he'd always had a tremor in his hand, and that tremor was his "friend", It kept him conscious; he told me of singing anything,

"No one should sign anything" he'd say.

He always turned misfortune into a laugh for me.

The complexities of the Medicare system in the United States are beyond the average human comprehension. Everyone knows this. Many lawyers, businesses, and companies specialize in ripping you off. Their claim is they can work through systems that you as the paying consumer will never totally understand. I believe this is true. It's all part of a big business, to try to understand the complexities so that you don't appear as an idiot. I don't mind appearing like an idiot. I've reached out to everyone I know for help and have been pleasantly surprised at the help I've gotten. I'm very lucky really. I also have an advisor, and now my friend called Les, he's there for me despite the fact he runs a major company in Utah, has forty people who call him almost daily, and works six days a week. He's a sounding board for me. I wonder if he knows how grateful I am for his help.

"Ask and you shall receive."

Matthew 7:7 in the bible

My lawyer, who is working for me, is gratis. I will call him My lawyer; Gregg, has helped me through the mire and the muck of this horrible

Medicare situation, the nursing home situation, and the ability to help Joseph. He's known Joseph for almost fifty years from New York days and has a deep consciousness few possess now. Lawyers in the USA are specialistic Deities. Your letter, email, or phone call will be tossed into the garbage, deleted, and shredded, but the Lawyers always get answered. Joseph needs a safe environment. This has not been easy. This has required endless letter writing, endless unanswered or unreturned phone calls, and endless stress. My Atty Gregg steps in every time to offer his advice and his brilliant letter writing.

One of the things I've noticed about myself now is, I have bags under my eyes. I look ten years older. I dream daily of returning to my beloved Beverly Hills, going to a plastic surgeon to have these bags removed, and becoming happy again. But I know realistically this is a far-off dream unless I have a miracle or win the lottery. Between those two things, the miracle is closer than the lottery. They say one in every 7 million people even buy a lottery ticket. I don't know if that's true, I know that most people that look like me never win the lottery, but that's irrelevant. Hope is all I have left. Enthusiasm is something I'm able to muster up, and so, every day I make my phone calls.

I've learned to beg. I'm quite good at it. I attended Acting classes at age eight, and finally, it's become useful. I'm a very good actress. I've gotten down on my knees and begged for a return phone call from the care facility that Joseph is in because that's the only way I will ever know anything about him. Recently, I was asked by his care facility to be on a 20-minute phone call with all his care providers, his nurses, his doctors, his psychiatrist, the dietician, and the activities director. All of it I considered to some degree to be passing bullshit, because he doesn't eat much of his food, he doesn't do activities, and he never will. They've asked me to consider imploring him to allow the nurses to weigh him, they have no idea how much he weighs. I was told he needs to get a Diabetes finger prick, which I know he'd never allow. He can't stand needles, but this too, is the system and I only have so much strength to fight daily. I simply cannot enter the ring all the time. A lot of my time is spent remembering to stroke the place that takes care of him, the nurses, and the administrators. It's all part of what I must do to keep him safe.

They weighed him the first day he came in, he was at 160 pounds, but he hasn't been eating for almost four months, no more than a few bites a day and he is skin and bones. It's hard to tell when you look at him what he was like before, but when I met him, 15 years ago, he weighed 200 pounds more. He was an average chubby, maybe even on the fat side, American. But in total good health, he lived the life of a rich man. He even had a bout of Gout, which is often referred to as a "rich man's disease." He ate three plus, four-course meals a day, and enjoyed every minute of the sunshine of Miami, FL. He would ride around on his golf cart with his little dog saying hello to his other 1 % ers. These Americans, are the ones who never know the side of what I'm talking about and who would have never predicted that this could have happened to him in any way, shape, or form.

I have risen to the challenges I now face, and I will succeed. I will make sure that Joseph is not put out on the curb and is not treated in an unjust way and after he passes on, which he will, I will continue to do this for others, not just the homeless, not just the indigent, not just the migrants, not just the refugees, but for all people. Fairness is an actuality that must be fought for, just like the democracy that we live in. Everybody needs help at one time or another. Everyone needs an advocate. This is my job now.

Although it's unpaid, it's worth my time.

I need a purpose in my life, my purpose was always Joseph, first, taking care of him as his girlfriend, now, taking care of him as his caregiver and his advocate, but soon I know that he will be gone from me, and I fear that I will become lost. I have lived the last 15 years of my life for this man, and I don't know what my future will look like without him. I do know that I refuse to become lost, I refuse to break, so I will continue fighting for the people who can't fight for themselves, and I will use this as my strength to keep moving forward. I know that I am a strong woman, and I will be able to face whatever life throws at me, this experience has taught me that,

I want to make Joseph proud.

I cherish this honor.

Chapter Twenty-Seven:

<><><><><><><><><><><><><><><><><><>

The Beginning of the End of Knowing Me

I always knew this day would possibly come before I felt ready to say goodbye, but now I've realized it's already here.

I'm not ready.

It's only been a week since Joseph said my name and a few months since he's been in the Nursing care facility in Los Angeles. I've been away from him in the physical for two months. I haven't held his hand in two months, and I swear that is something all patients need, love and a hand to hold. He has neither now in the flesh.

He's starting to not remember me and when he sees me on Facetime, like yesterday, he looks like he vaguely remembers me, and I say with extra love and patience in my voice,

"It's me, Sweetie, Cynthia". He makes a face. He's trying to remember.

"I know who you are," he states emphatically. He's agitated that I caught him not remembering, which actually makes me feel good. He still has that in him, a sense of pride in memory. But he doesn't really remember, and he doesn't want me to observe this in him. He knows my tone of voice, and my kindness to him. That he remembers. He loves that. But only so much of that can come through on a phone screen. He stares back at me, and I think he's fading in and out. I can feel this.

There are only so many more Facetimes we'll ever have.

My stomach is turning, and this dreaded feeling of losing him is too much to handle. I feel my tears welling up again, but he can't really focus now, and he doesn't see them.

I asked how his lunch was today.

"Wonderful," he states, and smiles. He's always detested and never ate the food in this place. The food is not fresh vegetables and fruit like he likes; it's processed and old. In his right mind, he would toss it out, but not now. His mind is no longer. This day is a day of horrors for me. It's the beginning of the near end.

This is the first time he's said he is enjoying it. I know it's because his body is starving to death, and I pray God sees this and takes him sooner rather than later. He's smiling and bored with our conversation after two minutes. I miss the days when he used to say,

"Talk to me more, don't hang up."

Now, nothing. He just stares at me and smiles. I smile back, but mine is tinged with sadness.

Now he's staring off to somewhere I've never been.

"Bye-bye, darling," I whisper into the phone.

He simply stares, not remembering what to say. After what seems like a long pause he says,

"Thank you."

I smile weakly.

My Heart Breaking, a single teardrop falling.

I hang up.

Chapter Twenty-Eight

<><><><><><><><><><><><><><><><>

The End of a Wonderful Chapter

This Dementia disease can affect anyone; it is more common than you know, and yet the research is usually about the patient, but what about the people who watch it happen?

The people like you.

The people like me.

Joseph was a love I never expected and never intended to have, but it is a love that I will always cherish. He made me feel like I was the only woman on this planet, and I adored him. I adored being his girlfriend, caring for him, pleasing him, and living my life for him. I enjoyed it because, in return, I felt complete.

I guess I was one of the lucky ones.

I lived a life with no cares; I lived a high life, a rich life, rich in experiences, rich in lifestyle, rich in material possessions. Having lunches with my girlfriends and elegant meals with my boyfriend, I would never have thought my life would change. I had settled on it being this way until the book of my life ended and the curtain closed, but that wasn't my destiny.

The universe wasn't through with me yet.

My wake-up call came when Joseph was in hospital, and my luxury lifestyle came crashing down.

I now fight for my survival. I will keep myself off the streets, out of the homeless encampments and I heavily rely on the kindness of others to help me through. I fight daily to make sure that the man who took care of me for 15 years isn't left to disappear in a transient home. I have had to dig deep within myself to create a new life for myself and Enzo and figure out ways that I can make money so I can rebuild my crumbling existence. I must fight with the government agencies for the poor to keep Joseph housed and cared for, I have to deal with the reality that I, too, am practically BROKE, and I have to watch my boyfriend, this mental genius, disappear before my eyes.

I am terrified of the day he doesn't remember me, yet I know that day will come soon.

I guess I know my story is quite bizarre. Last year, I lived in a New York Upper East Side, an elegant apartment with a doorman, elevator operator, and 24/7 white glove service, living a lifestyle with a boyfriend who adored me. Now, as we reach the final months, only a year later, I am in a cottage in Pennsylvania at my brother's house, trying to create and rebuild my broken life, alone, while preparing to say goodbye to my King of New York, my best friend, my boyfriend Joseph.

I am trying my hardest to stay positive and I am putting all my attention into being Joseph's advocate, I guess this is distracting me from my reality. I have always loved caring for Joseph, and in his final months, I will continue to do this. I am not prepared to even think of what will happen when he has gone, what my life will become, where will I place my energy then?

Continuing to meditate and pray is my only option, hoping the creativity within me will spark a new project to keep me busy. Putting my energy into helping people less fortunate and being an advocate for those who may need it will become my passion. I refuse to break even though the universe has thrown everything at me to make that so.

I may be broke, but I will not be broken.

In mere months I have lost everything, my riches, my lifestyle, my home, my friends, and my best friend and love, Joseph.

This has been my "Wake Up Call."

But this is not my ending. This is just a new beginning.

This just may become my reinvention.

I still speak to Joseph when I can via FaceTime, when I can get a nurse to facilitate the call and so far, he still knows my face, even if it is vaguely. I still fill in nursing facility forms daily and fight the bureaucracy; I still meditate and pray.

That woman who began this year is no more the same person, but in her place is a woman filled with strength and appreciation for what is important in life.

What remains in her life and what is yet to be discovered?

I can see Joseph fading before my eyes, his sparkle weakening by the day, I hold on to the fact he still knows my face and dread the day that he doesn't. I know it is near.

I realize my story isn't unique, and I know that I am not the only person who has experienced this crumbling of a life you didn't know was on such a short timescale, but this is MY story, and I hope it brings you what it needs to bring you.

Whatever that may be.

This is a story about strength. I would be lying if I said that this past year hasn't been anything but hell, but it has made me a more resilient woman. I now know what I am made of. I hope it brings you courage, the courage to stay the course, the courage to move forward, and a true appreciation of life, no matter the circumstances.

To Joseph,

I love you, and I thank you, for the life you gave me and the love you filled me up with. I will be here until the end and until the curtain closes on your final act.

Just like I promised.

Chapter Twenty-Nine:

◇◇◆◆◆◆◆◆◆◆◆◆◆◇◇

The Dreaded Finale

I was thinking about the Blue Moon, tonight. It always inspires me, filling me with hope and determination. It's been said it's a time to honor the endings in life to begin anew.

No matter what, it's a catalyst of the unknown.

Little did I know tonight would be that time of my foreseeing.

Irina, the Social Aide at the Nursing Care Facility agreed to facilitate my Facetime with Joseph. I had a feeling she knew something I did not. She was acting out in her cheery self,

when I said,

"He can only speak a few words now, but I want to see him, if only for a couple of minutes."

"Of course, Dear," she said. I could see her face on Facetime, and although she was her ever-pleasant self, there was some trepidation.

As she walked into his room, I felt relief, if only for a moment. He was lying on his back eating a piece of fruit. It was messy, dripping on his hands and bed sheet. His usual serviette was nowhere in sight. I wondered what fruit it was. No matter. Nothing mattered in this moment except for the fact we were together even though on video.

She held her phone in front of his face, and he stared at me, at it, then at her.

He was lost in the moment, lost in a space that I'd never been to with him.

"I love you, Joseph," I offered up in hopes of a return thought from him.

He always recognized my face and always smiled at hearing my voice.

Now, he stares at me.

Nothing.

"I miss you, Sweetheart, "I uttered softly, and with tears in my eyes, I'd hope he couldn't see.

I don't think he's able to focus now on anyone, or anything.

He stares at me on the screen.

He's trying to form a word from the corner of his mouth. He's remembering me now.

I can see his lips moving ever so slowly

"I miss you," he whispers, barely audible.

It's as though I've learned to read lips, learned by loving him, to read his mind, learned by looking into the soul of a man I spent fifteen years with, learned by the light in his eyes,

He's departing now. This is the finale of what I've been dreading, and now I'm living it.

He's leaving me now, never to return.

And I know that he knows.

As his eyes wander off, I feel the loss of my best friend as a death, but he still breathes as we wait for his final departure.

The final blue moon lights the sky as he
passes through the veil.
His brilliant mind laid to rest.
He resides in 'The Court of Kings' at
Hillside Memorial in Los Angeles.
The closing of his book.

www.ingramcontent.com/pod-product-compliance
Lightning Source LLC
Chambersburg PA
CBHW071327120626
46546CB00002B/474